CRIMINAL PSYCHOLOGY
& PERSONALITY PROFILING

SOLVING CRIMES WITH SCIENCE:
Forensics

CRIMINAL PSYCHOLOGY & PERSONALITY PROFILING

Joan Esherick

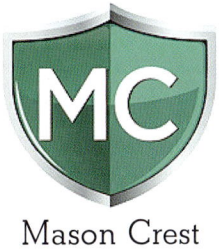

Mason Crest

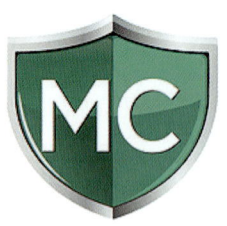

Mason Crest
450 Parkway Drive, Suite D
Broomall, PA 19008
www.masoncrest.com

Printed and bound in the United States of America.

9 8 7 6 5 4 3 2

Series ISBN: 978-1-4222-2861-6
ISBN: 978-1-4222-2863-0

ebook ISBN: 978-1-4222-8949-5

The Library of Congress has cataloged the
hardcopy format(s) as follows:

Library of Congress Cataloging-in-Publication Data

Esherick, Joan.
  Criminal psychology & personality profiling / Joan Esherick.
    p. cm. — (Solving crimes with science, forensics)
  Audience: 012.
  Audience: Grades 7 to 8.
  Includes bibliographical references and index.
  ISBN 978-1-4222-2863-0 (hardcover) — ISBN 978-1-4222-2861-6 (series) — ISBN 978-1-4222-8949-5 (ebook)
  1. Criminal psychology—Juvenile literature. 2. Criminal behavior, Prediction of—Juvenile literature. 3. Criminal profilers—Juvenile literature. 4. Forensic sciences—Juvenile literature. I. Title. II. Title: Criminal psychology and personality profiling.
  HV6080.E795 2014
  614.15—dc23
                            2013006932

Produced by Vestal Creative Services.
www.vestalcreative.com

Contents

Introduction

By Jay A. Siegel, Ph.D.
Director, Forensic and Investigative Sciences Program
Indiana University, Purdue University, Indianapolis

It seems like every day the news brings forth another story about crime in the United States. Although the crime rate has been slowly decreasing over the past few years (due perhaps in part to the aging of the population), crime continues to be a very serious problem. Increasingly, the stories we read that involve crimes also mention the role that forensic science plays in solving serious crimes. Sensational crimes provide real examples of the power of forensic science. In recent years there has been an explosion of books, movies, and TV shows devoted to forensic science and crime investigation. The wondrously successful *CSI* TV shows have spawned a major increase in awareness of and interest in forensic science as a tool for solving crimes. *CSI* even has its own syndrome: the "*CSI* Effect," wherein jurors in real cases expect to hear testimony about science such as fingerprints, DNA, and blood spatter because they saw it on TV.

The unprecedented rise in the public's interest in forensic science has fueled demands by students and parents for more educational programs that teach the applications of science to crime. This started in colleges and universities but has filtered down to high schools and middle schools. Even elementary school students now learn how science is used in the criminal justice system. Most educators agree that this developing interest in forensic science is a good thing. It has provided an excellent opportunity to teach students science—and they have fun learning it! Forensic science is an ideal vehicle for teaching science for several reasons. It is truly multidisciplinary; practically every field of science has forensic applications. Successful forensic scientists must be good problem solvers and critical thinkers. These are critical skills that all students need to develop.

In all of this rush to implement forensic science courses in secondary schools throughout North America, the development of grade-appropriate resources that help guide students and teachers is seriously lacking. This new series: *Solving Crimes With Science: Forensics* is important and timely. Each book in the series contains a concise, age-appropriate discussion of one or more areas of forensic science.

Students are never too young to begin to learn the principles and applications of science. Forensic science provides an interesting and informative way to introduce scientific concepts in a way that grabs and holds the students' attention. *Solving Crimes With Science: Forensics* promises to be an important resource in teaching forensic science to students twelve to eighteen years old.

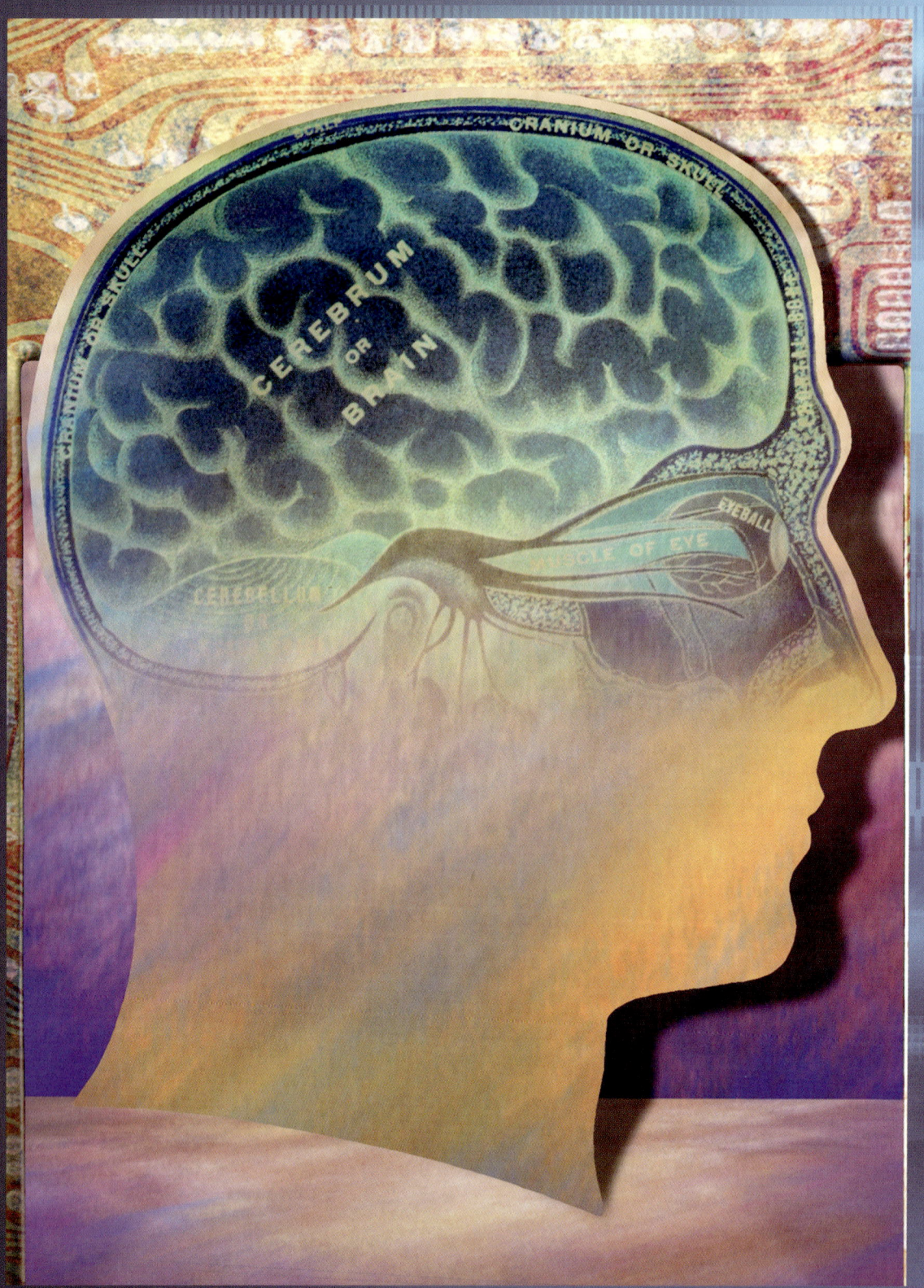

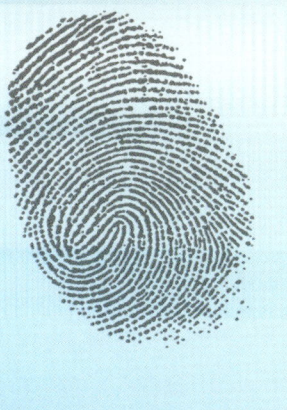

WHAT IS CRIMINAL PSYCHOLOGY?

In Sacramento, California, for no apparent reason, an unknown assailant shoots and kills a middle-aged man on the street. Less than a year later, the same assailant uses a knife to brutally murder a young pregnant woman in her bedroom. Three days later he strikes again, this time killing a thirty-six-year-old woman, her six-year-old son, and an adult male friend of the family, all in the woman's home. The murderer shoots his victims with a .22 caliber handgun or rifle. The killer also kidnaps the woman's twenty-two-month-old nephew and steals the visiting friend's station wagon, which is later abandoned near the crime scene and recovered by authorities.

Police know they have a dangerous criminal on their hands, perhaps a serial murderer. They seek outside help to more quickly solve the crime. They hire a consultant who provides these clues about the suspect:

- If the suspect owns a car, it will be a "wreck, with fast-food wrappers in the back, and rust throughout."
- He's a white male; 25 to 27 years old; thin; undernourished in appearance.
- The killer lives near the victims.
- He's a loner, lives alone, and is unemployed.
- He has a history of mental illness.
- His home will be "slovenly and unkempt."
- He lives within a half-mile to a mile of the abandoned station wagon.
- Before he started killing, this man probably burglarized homes near the murder sites.

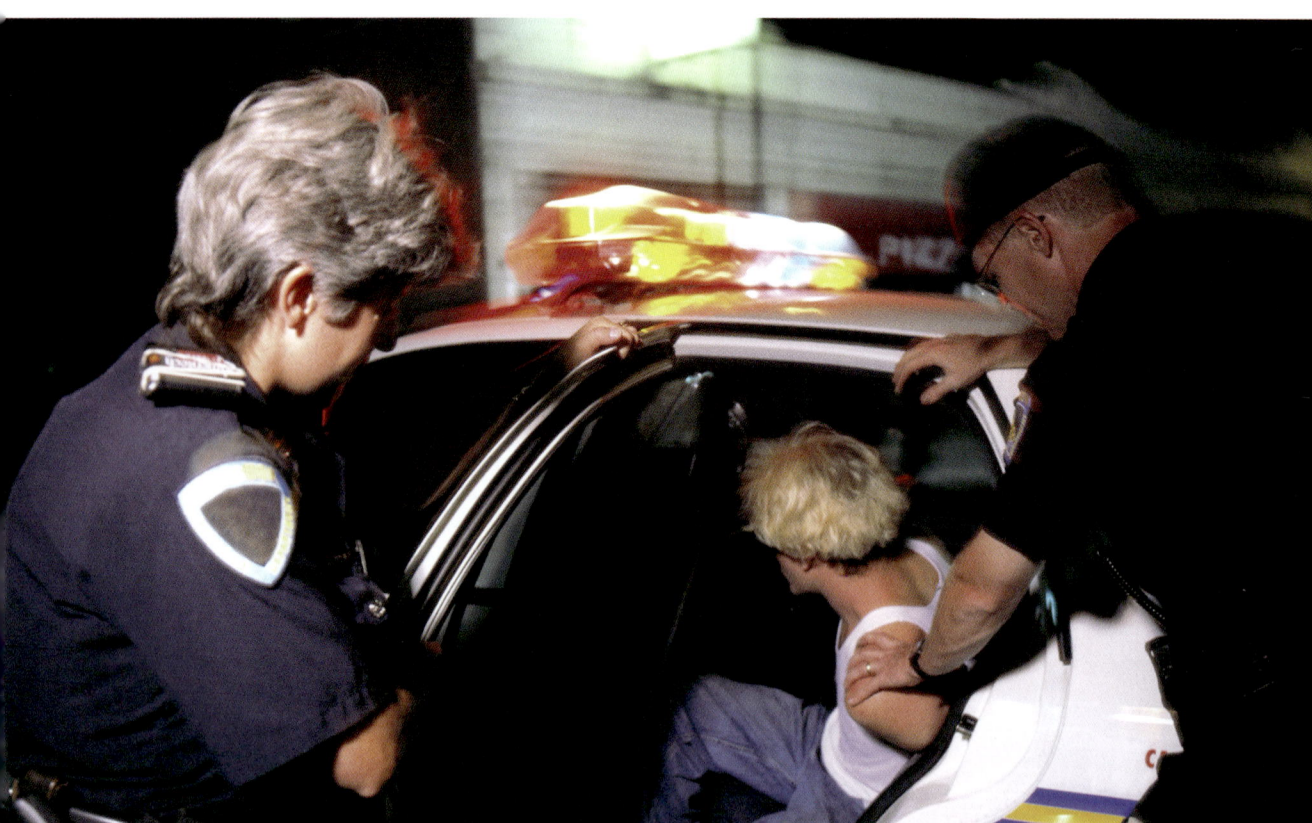

Psychological profiles of criminals can lead investigators to an arrest.

Armed with this information, police canvas the area within a half-mile radius of the abandoned stolen car, interviewing the hundreds of people who live there. One woman recalls speaking to a man whose appearance shocked her: "disheveled, cadaverously thin, bloody sweat-shirt, yellowed crust around his mouth, sunken eyes." Because she knew the man years earlier in high school, she is able to name him: Richard Trenton Chase.

Just as the consultant suggested, Chase's apartment is located less than a block from the abandoned stolen car. His vehicle, a truck, is parked nearby. Inside the beat-up old truck, again as the consultant had predicted, police find rags, trash, beer cans, empty milk cartons, and discarded newspapers. The vehicle is in poor condition. They also find a twelve-inch (30-centimeter) butcher knife and boots spattered with blood.

Again consistent with the consultant's information, the suspect's apartment is a complete mess. Investigators also find evidence of horrific activities there: three food blenders with blood in them, bloody clothing, newspaper articles about the first killing, and a refrigerator containing dishes with human remains.

Police arrest Richard Trenton Chase, who is later convicted of six murders and sentenced to die in California's gas chamber. He commits suicide in his death-row cell before he can be executed.

These events occurred in 1980. The case required help beyond the bounds of typical law enforcement. Investigators used profiling, one aspect of criminal psychology, to solve the case.

CASE STUDY:
A PSYCHIC DETECTIVE

In Staunton, Virginia, a masked rapist assaults five women and is suspected of assaulting several more in the area. With no physical descriptions to help them identify the perpetrator, police can do little to solve the crimes. Without leads or any new clues, they aren't sure where to turn. Then a consultant provides this information about the rapist:

- He has a scar on his leg.
- He is skilled with mechanical things.
- He apologizes to his victims.
- People view him as a "nice guy."
- He wears a green uniform.
- He's been in prison before.
- He lives near a theater in a brick building at the bottom of a hill.
- He drives a truck that "goes round and round."

The Staunton Police Department's consultant then accurately describes how the rapist entered the crime scenes and where the rapist waited for his victims. She provides this information without the police giving her any details of the crimes.

In a later investigation of another crime, police arrest a suspect whose description bears an uncanny resemblance to the information earlier provided by the consultant about the serial rapist. Because of the similarities between the man they have in custody and the consultant's description, police question him about the rapes. The man, James B. Robinson, eventually confesses to the sexual assaults.

The consultant's information is amazingly on target: Robinson drives a cement truck for a living (a truck with a revolving mixer that "goes round and round"); his leg is scarred; he claims to feel badly about the attacks and, indeed, apologized to his victims; he lives across the street from the Dixie Theater in a brick apartment building at the base of a steep hill; and he has a prison record.

Under a plea-bargain agreement, Robinson pleads guilty to five rapes and sixteen other felonies and is sentenced to twenty-one concurrent twenty-year prison sentences.

Although this case might sound like the work of a profiler, it's not. The consultant in this case was a psychic detective. Psychic detectives generally have little or no training in crime science, law enforcement, psychiatry, or psychology. They use what they call their "psychic abilities" to "sense" things about a crime victim or perpetrator. They rely on feelings, instincts, and visions to solve crimes. Psychic detectives describe their "gifts" as supernatural, and most law enforcement officers cannot explain how these seers do what they seem to do. But they are not profilers or criminal psychologists, and little or no science or education is involved.

Criminal Psychology: Not What You Think

When the average person hears the terms "criminal psychology" and "profiling," he imagines several things. First, he often assumes these words refer to the same people, jobs, or procedures. They do not. He might think criminal psychologists and profilers identify unknown suspects by name. They don't. They can't.

Much common understanding of the world of criminal psychology comes from what is portrayed in print media or on television. Shows like NBC's *Profiler* (1996–2000), CBS's *CSI: Crime Scene Investigation* (2000–), and NBC's *Medium* (2005–2011), though entertaining, blur the lines between fact and fantasy.

Consider the late 1990s hit series Profiler, for example. The main character in this investigative crime drama was Dr. Samantha Waters, played by Ally Walker. Media trailers and reviews alternately described her as a "forensic psychologist" or a "psychic detective." Which was she? Or was she both? Weekly episodes portrayed the investigator as a scientist who used physical evidence and laboratory methods, along with her powers of observation, her understanding of criminal psychology, and the graphic supernatural visions that appeared in her mind throughout the show to catch criminals. She acted as a criminal investigator, psychologist, and psychic. For this television program and others like it, science and the supernatural went hand in hand.

Real-world criminal psychology is very different. When it comes to studying and solving crime, authentic criminal psychologists and profilers are very different entities. Here's how they differ:

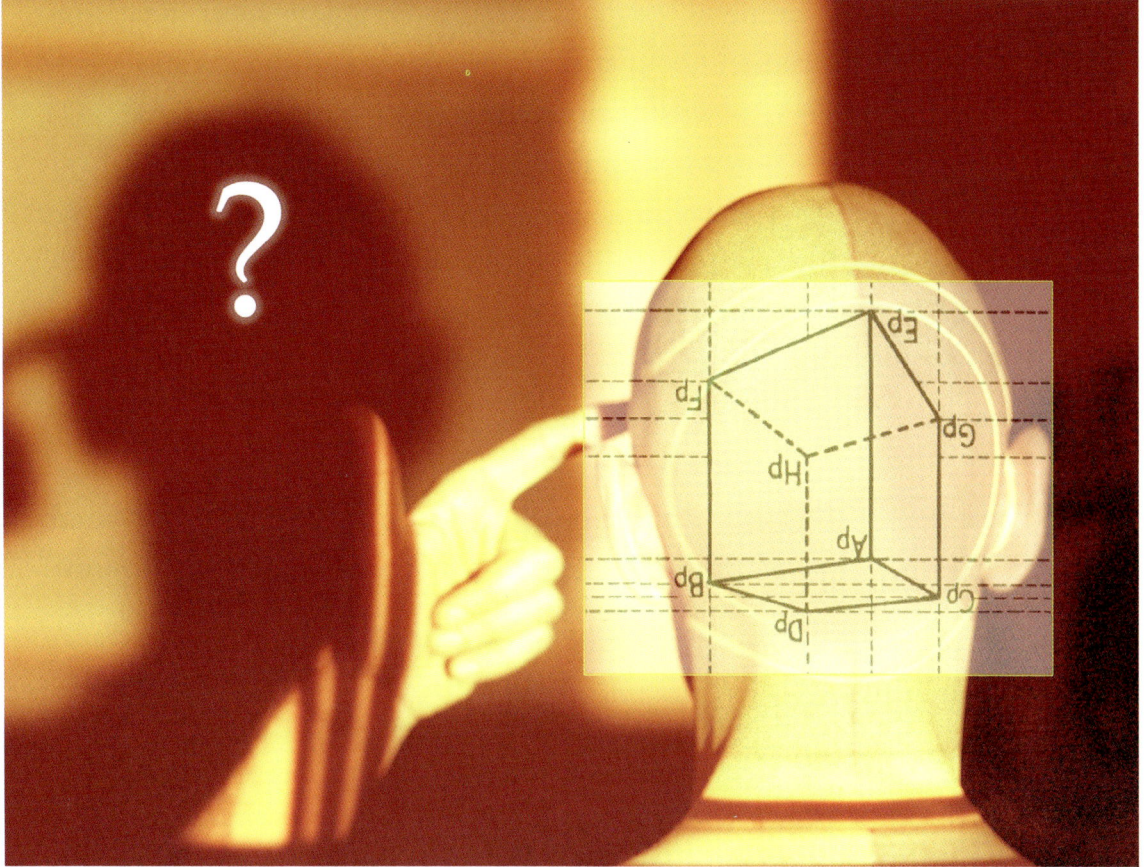

Profiles outline a criminal's general traits and how that criminal might act.

- *Criminal psychologists* study the minds and behaviors of criminals and others associated with crime in order to understand how and why they operate the way they do and to identify certain patterns of behavior. These professionals usually earn advanced degrees in psychology, psychiatry, criminology, or law enforcement, and they base much of their work on experience, interviews, and firsthand observance of people who commit and are affected by crime.

What Is Criminal Psychology?

- *Profilers* are criminal psychologists who study hard facts and targeted information about specific criminals and their crime scenes and then summarize what they discover into general behavioral traits, patterns, and characteristics that fit the known facts. Based on this information, they develop a partial description of how the suspect would most likely act, what his personality would most likely be like, and what his past might have involved according to the behavior he displays in the crimes. Profilers are only one kind of criminal psychologist; there are many more.

In the scenario that opened this chapter, the Sacramento Police Department called in behavioral scientist Robert Ressler, the founder and former

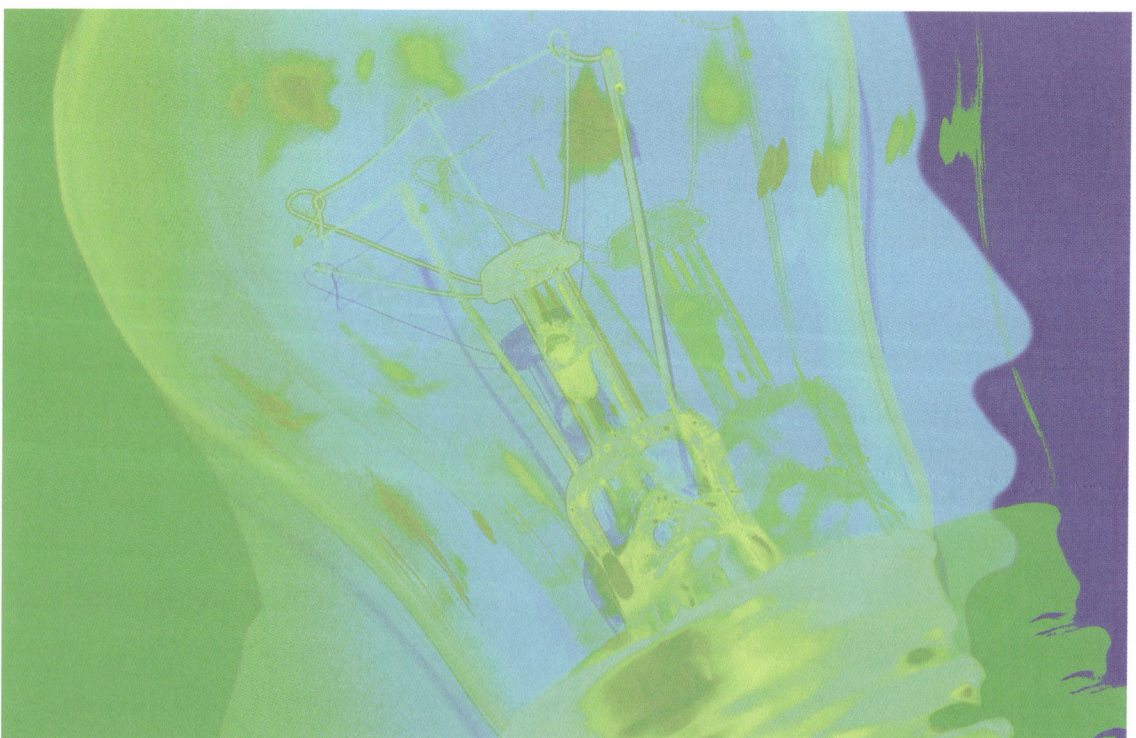

Criminal psychology is a tool investigators can use to help identify a suspect. It can shed light on the criminal mind.

Fast Fact

In the sixteenth century and for hundreds of years after, physicians and law enforcement officials believed that a person's physical traits (forehead, mouth, eyes, teeth, nose, and hair) revealed whether he had a criminal nature. This practice was called physiognomy.

director of the FBI's Violent Criminal Apprehension Program. As a highly educated expert on serial killers and sexual homicides, he was able to accurately profile the offender based on his study of the crime scenes, the nature of the crimes, and his studies of the criminal mind and other criminals.

Criminal Psychology: Relatively New

Though recent interest in forensic sciences (any science used for the purpose of law) has sparked public interest in the workings of a criminal mind, the field of study called criminal psychology has been around for a long time. In fact, one textbook still used today, *Criminal Psychology: A Manual for Judges, Practitioners, and Students,* was written by Hans Gross and originally published in 1911.

Even though philosophers began using the term "psychology" in the seventeenth century to describe how the mind influenced behavior, it wasn't until the twentieth century that most people who studied crime looked

An 1895 Listing of Criminals' Physical Traits

Nineteenth-century Italian professor of forensic medicine Cesare Lombroso felt he could identify criminals by their physical characteristics. After studying over 6,000 convicted criminals, he determined the following:

- Assassins have prominent jaws, widely separated cheekbones, thick dark hair, and pale skin.
- Assailants have rounded skulls, wide foreheads, and long hands.
- Thieves have abnormal skull sizes, thick hair, and full beards.
- Rapists have short hands, narrow foreheads, and abnormal noses.
- Arsonists have long arms and legs, small heads, and are underweight.
- Pickpockets are tall with long hands, dark hair, and scanty beards.

Recent research doesn't back up Lombroso's findings!

for reasons beyond the physical or spiritual to explain criminal behavior. As understanding of the mind and its workings grew in the early 1900s, criminologists began to realize that criminal behavior finds its source not in physical abnormalities or spiritual influences, but rather in the mind.

As its name implies, criminal psychology examines the minds, attitudes, and actions of people who commit crimes, their victims, witnesses to crimes, and people in law enforcement. Criminal psychologists study people who commit or are impacted by crimes to understand what makes them behave as they do. As Gross defines it, criminal psychology is a "***pragmatic*** applied psychology [that deals] with all states of mind that might possibly be involved in the determination and judgment of crime."

To achieve this level of understanding, criminal psychologists study several things about people: general psychology (the study of the mind and behavior of individuals and how they relate to others); relationships and how they influence the mind and behavior; the dynamics of people's pasts and their influences today; and people's mannerisms, intellectual processes, intelligence, emotions, and memories. Criminal psychologists also study other topics and issues beyond the individual: law enforcement behaviors, how interviews are handled, how suspects are questioned,

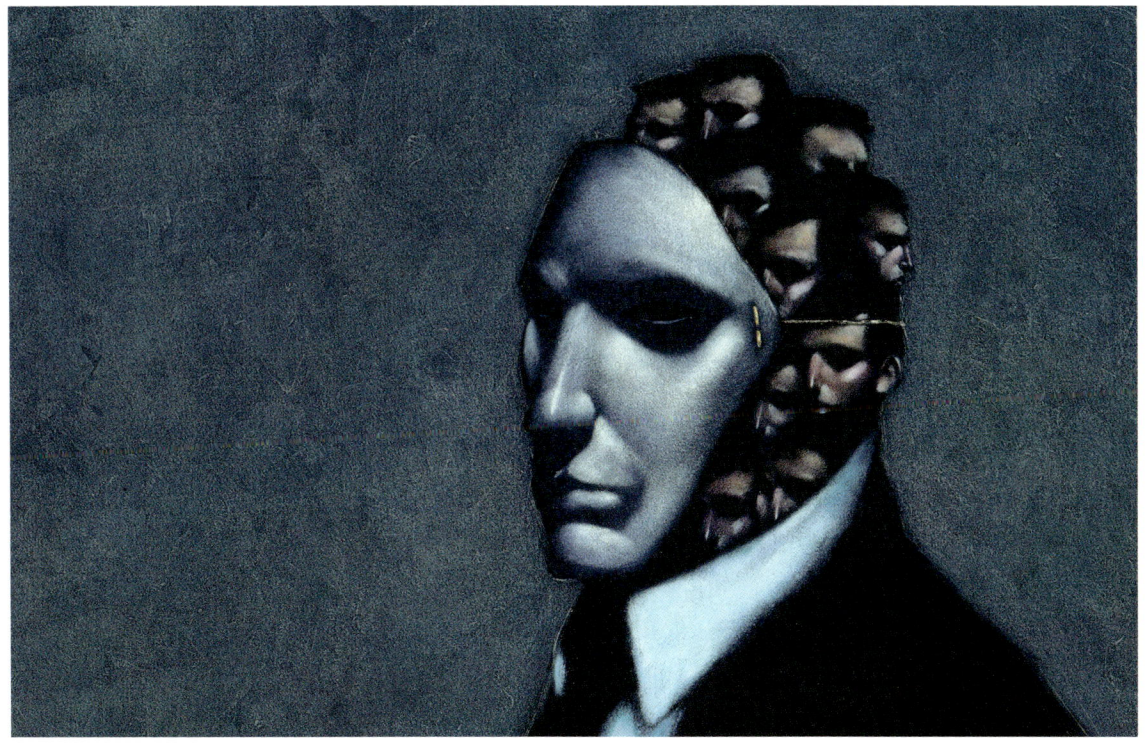

Criminal psychologists attempt to see beyond the mask a criminal wears.

What Is Criminal Psychology?   **19**

The Mad Bomber

Between 1940 and 1956 an unknown assailant left over fifty bombs in public places all over New York City. Called the "Mad Bomber," the offender wrote letters to newspapers describing his reasons for terrorizing the city, but he eluded police for sixteen years until detectives consulted Dr. James A. Brussels, a psychiatrist who worked extensively with criminals.

After studying the evidence, including the contents of letters the bomber had sent, Brussels described the criminal: "Single man between 40 and 50 years old, introvert. Unsocial, but not antisocial. Skilled mechanic. . . . Moral. Honest. Not interested in women. High school graduate. Expert in civil or military [law]. Religious. . . . Present or former Consolidated Edison [a New York City utility company] worker. Probable case of progressive paranoia."

The psychiatrist also told police the man they were looking for would be well built and cleanly shaved, would live with an older female relative, probably in Connecticut, and would wear neatly buttoned double-breasted suits.

When the Mad Bomber, George Metesky, was finally arrested, Brussels's description matched him almost perfectly: he lived in Connecticut with his two elderly half-sisters; he was middle-aged and single; he was a solidly built, well-groomed, clean-shaven man; he had once worked as a skilled laborer for Consolidated Edison; and when police brought him in, he wore a double-breasted suit, neatly buttoned.

courtroom dynamics, the stressors involved in witnessing or giving testimony about crime, communication styles, gender influences, the art of persuasion, and a host of other factors that can influence how a person acts in a police interrogation room or courtroom either as witness or suspected offender.

All these topics fall under the broad category of behavioral sciences. These aren't *objective* sciences in the way mathematics or chemistry are; they are *subjective* sciences, meaning they depend more on interpretation, observation, opinion, and perception than on formulas, equations, or physical laws.

No medical, mathematical, or scientific formula exists to determine that a person will act a certain way—not the way medical tests for diabetes can determine that the body will handle sugars in a certain way. But thousands of hours of observations about people and how they behave can help criminal psychologists hypothesize what a person will *most likely* do in certain circumstances or how an individual will *most likely* act as a result of certain experiences. Criminal psychologists cannot guarantee outcomes the way a mathematician can guarantee that two plus two will always equal four. But because human behavior is somewhat predictable, criminal psychologists can deal in likelihoods. Take serial killers, for example.

Serial Killers: An Example of How Criminal Psychology Works

No definitive measure exists today that will determine if someone will become a serial killer. But after studying hundreds of serial killers (their his-

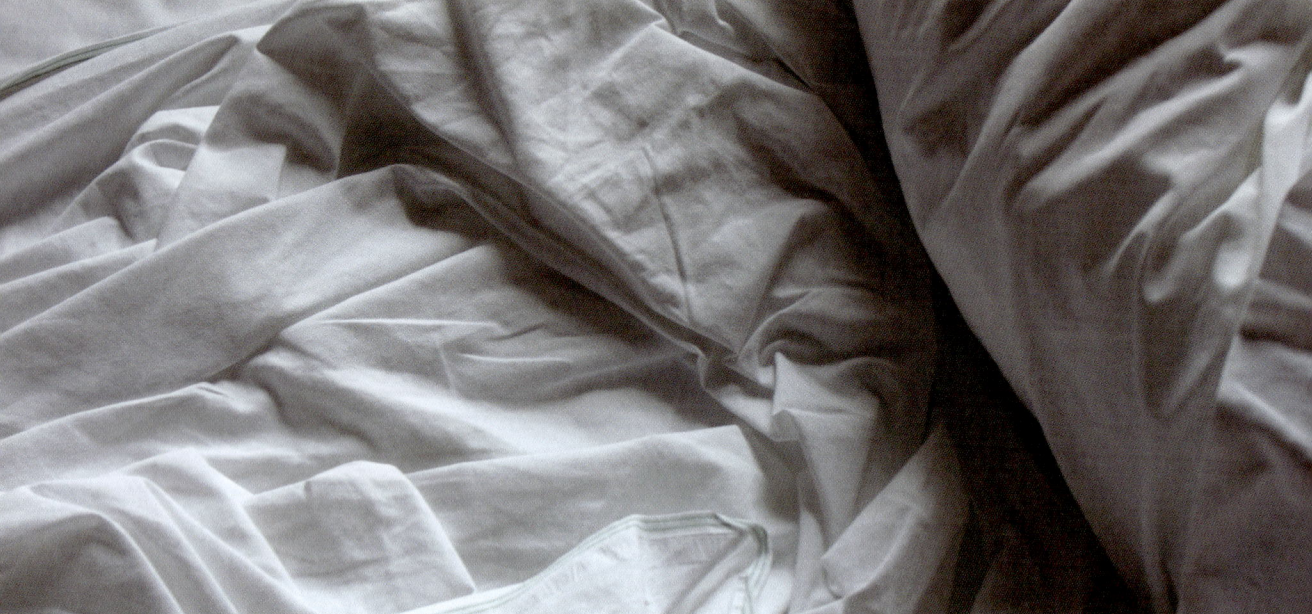

Bed wetting during childhood is a common symptom in serial killers.

tories, their childhoods, and their responses to interview questions over decades of time), criminal psychologists have learned that serial killers have certain things in common: in the United States and Canada they tend to be single, Caucasian males; they usually have above-average IQs; despite their intelligence, most did not do well in school; most come from deeply troubled families; and most show signs of psychiatric problems from very young ages. In fact, criminal psychologists and mental health officials have come up with three key warning signs, something they call the psychopathological triad, that virtually all serial killers interviewed held in common as children: they tended to wet their beds until late in childhood, they liked to set fires, and they enjoyed torturing small animals.

While not every child who experiences enuresis (bedwetting), pyromania (fire-starting), and **precocious** sadism (childhood delight in torturing animals) grows up to become a serial killer, children who demonstrate these traits are *more likely* than someone without those characteristics to do so. This psychopathological triad may not expose a serial killer the way X-rays reveal a broken bone, but it does give criminal psychologists and law enforcement officials a significant clue and a predictor about a person's potential for future violence.

Much of criminal psychology and profiling works this way: the criminal psychologist compares a criminal's or witness's current behaviors with those of thousands who previously experienced similar situations and then makes educated predictions about how the individual is most likely to behave based on what others like him have done before. More often than not, these predictions are accurate.

The ability to make these assessments about people comes from years of education, training, experience, and observation. No magic or psychic visions are involved—just hard work, knowledge, and practical application. The best criminal psychologists are usually those with the most experience in the field.

As you might suspect, having this ability to assess and predict behavior can come in quite handy not only for solving crime, but also for other aspects of criminology and the criminal justice system: picking juries, preparing witnesses for testimony, giving testimony about a person's likelihood to commit crime, interviewing suspects, and so on. As we see in the media, some criminal psychologists become experts in profiling to solve crime, as did the criminal psychologist who helped the Sacramento Police in this chapter's opening case. But many more help in other areas of the legal and justice systems by advising police, counseling lawyers, offering input to judges and juries, training others, and educating the public.

Though criminal psychology may be a subjective science, criminal psychologists serve in many roles, providing tangible help to police officers, jurists, judges, lawyers, analysts, and average citizens all over the world.

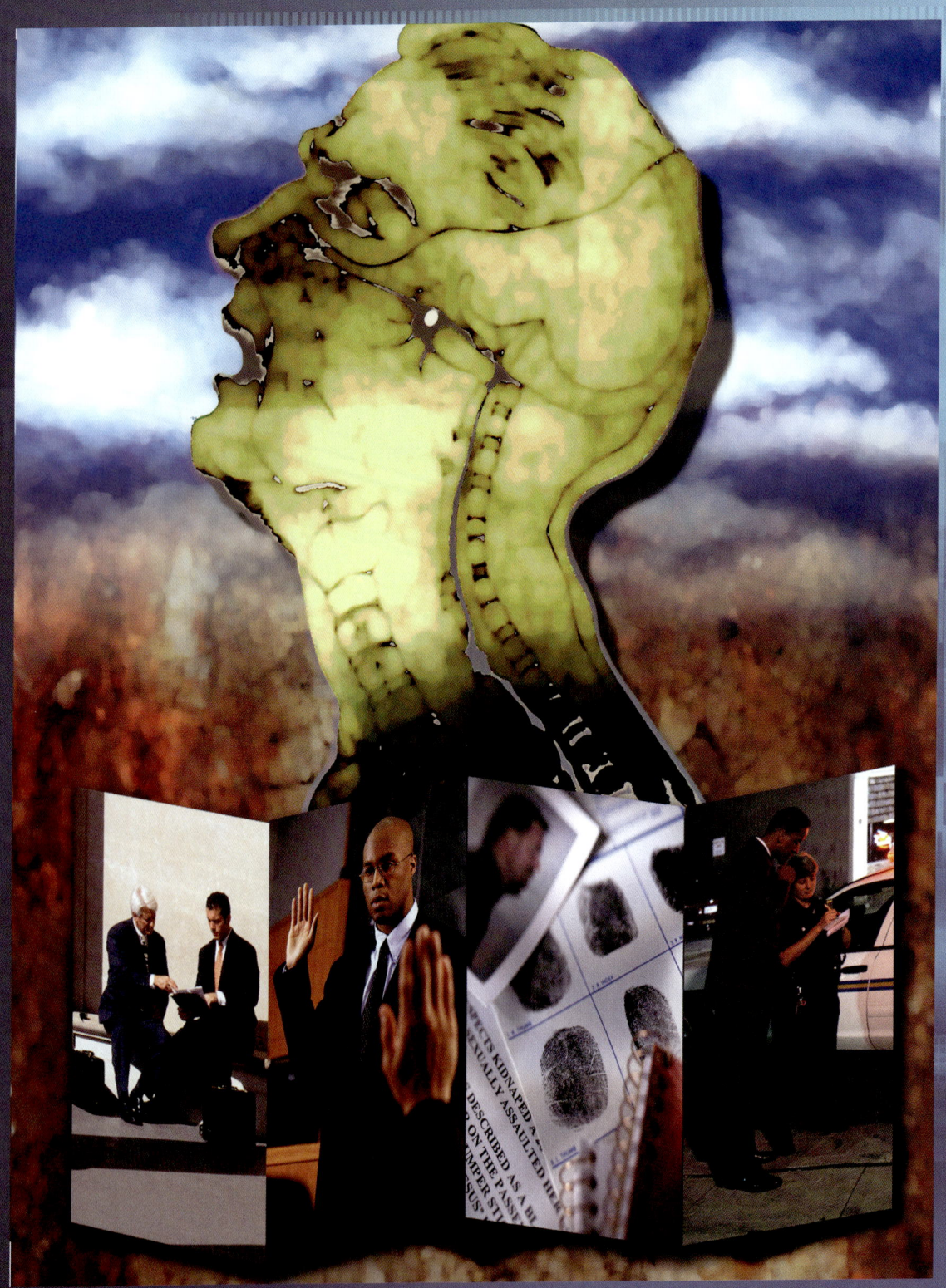

2

THE MANY ROLES OF A CRIMINAL PSYCHOLOGIST

1. A woman testifies for the prosecution in a New York courtroom to establish whether a defendant is faking mental illness.

2. A retired professional consults with San Diego County's deputy district attorney about a series of crimes to determine if they are linked.

3. A doctor takes the stand as an expert witness in a high-profile murder trial to convince the jury to spare a defendant from the death penalty.

4. A U.S. law enforcement official gives counsel to Canadian prosecutors about how to examine an accused murderer when he takes the witness stand at his trial.

5. Researchers in Vancouver use computer programs to evaluate crime locations to develop an idea of where the perpetrators live and where they will most likely strike again.

6. A former state commissioner of public safety lectures forensics students about his view of the evidence in a famous unsolved murder.

Who are these people, and what do they have in common? All of them serve in one capacity or another as criminal psychologists.

- First on the list is Barbara Kirwin, Ph.D., author of *The Mad, the Bad, and the Innocent*, a forensic psychologist who often provides expert testimony about a defendant's sanity for courts in New York State.
- Second is Roy Hazelwood, the former FBI profiler who provided analysis to San Diego County's deputy district attorney that linked a series of crimes in 1992 and 1993 to the Pacific Beach Rapist. The links he established between the crimes ultimately resulted in the rapist's conviction.

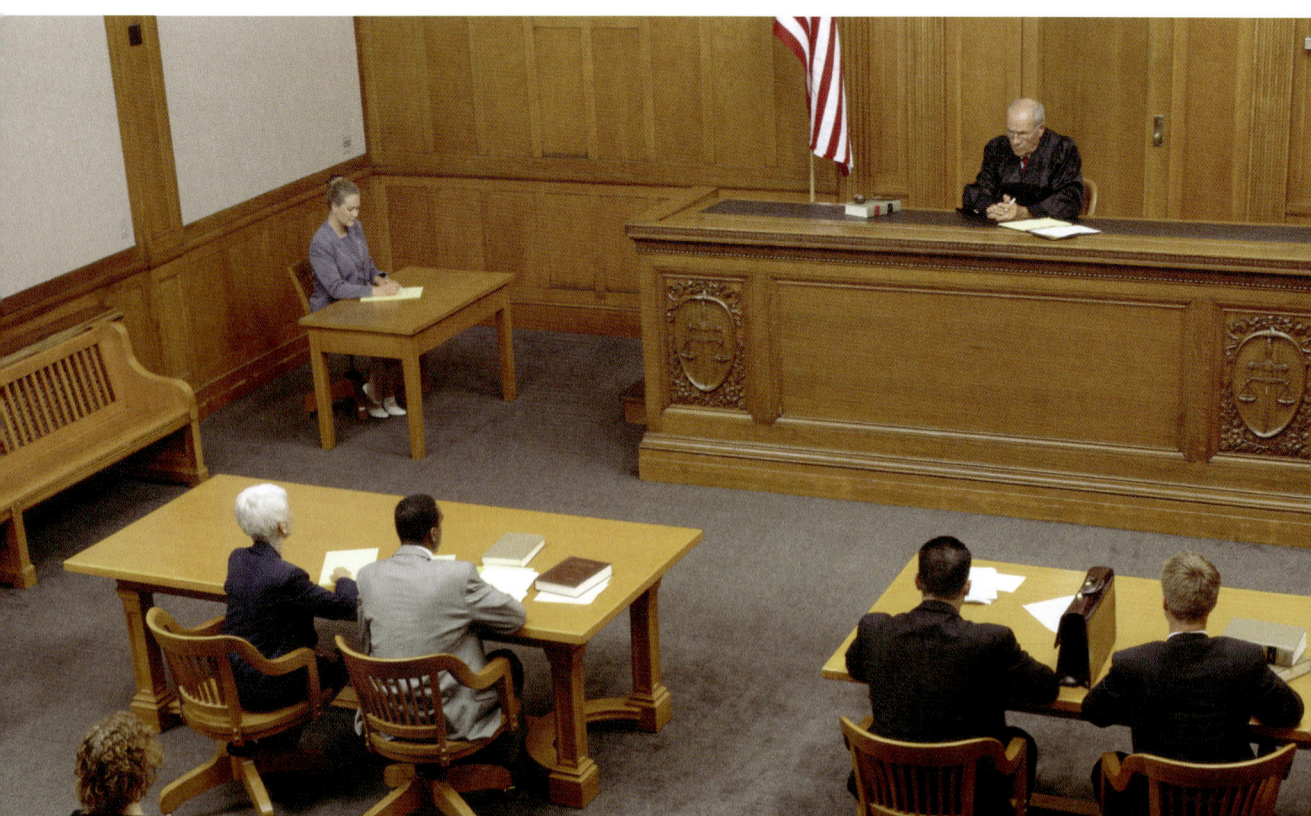

Criminal psychology has played a role in many high-profile court cases.

- Third is psychiatrist Helen Morrison, M.D., who testified in serial-murderer John Wayne Gacy's trial. Despite her testimony that he was insane, the jury did not accept Gacy's insanity defense and sentenced him to death. He died by lethal injection on May 10, 1994.

- Following Morrison on the list is John Douglas, a former FBI agent and renowned expert in personality profiling and criminal analysis. In this situation, the Crown attorney (Canada) asked Douglas to help Toronto prosecutors develop a strategy to agitate accused murderer Tien Poh Su on the witness stand, allowing the jury to see his extreme emotional responses. Douglas provided a strategy, the defendant became extremely upset when he testified, and the jury convicted him of murder.

- In the fifth case, Dr. Kim Rosso, a detective inspector in Vancouver, British Columbia, worked with colleagues to develop a "criminal geographic targeting" (CGT) computer system that can be used to indicate the probable location of a serial offender's home base or "anchor point"—often the general area in which he lives.

- The last situation involved Dr. Henry Lee, founder of the University of New Haven's forensic science program. He was concluding a special lecture series on famous crimes, and his last lecture concerned the *plausibility* of various theories about the death of Colorado child beauty queen JonBenet Ramsey. To date, that case remains unsolved.

In these situations, each individual served in a specific role as a criminal psychologist. Each one's expertise helped law enforcement officials, court officials, or those training to become so.

Ultimately, that is the primary role of a criminal psychologist: to support others in the law enforcement and criminal justice systems. The criminal psychologist most often serves as one tool in the varied toolboxes of crimi-

Careers in Criminal Psychology: More Varied Than You Think!

A criminal-psychology major in college prepares students for many potential careers. Most careers, however, also require postcollege education, training, or graduate degrees:

counselor

therapist

psychiatrist

criminal psychologist

crime-scene analyst

crime-scene investigator

police officer

detective

investigator

federal agent (FBI, CIA, DEA,
 Secret Service, CSIS, RCMP)

homeland security advisor

corrections officer

parole or probation officer

lawyer

social worker

court advocate

mental health worker

private consultant

author

educator (teacher, professor,
 trainer)

public servant

nologists, law enforcement officials, lawyers, judges, and others who seek to address crime and criminal behavior.

Because criminal psychologists play a supporting part in the overall crime drama, their roles vary. Their expertise can help police, lawyers, courts, jury consultants, witnesses, and students in several ways.

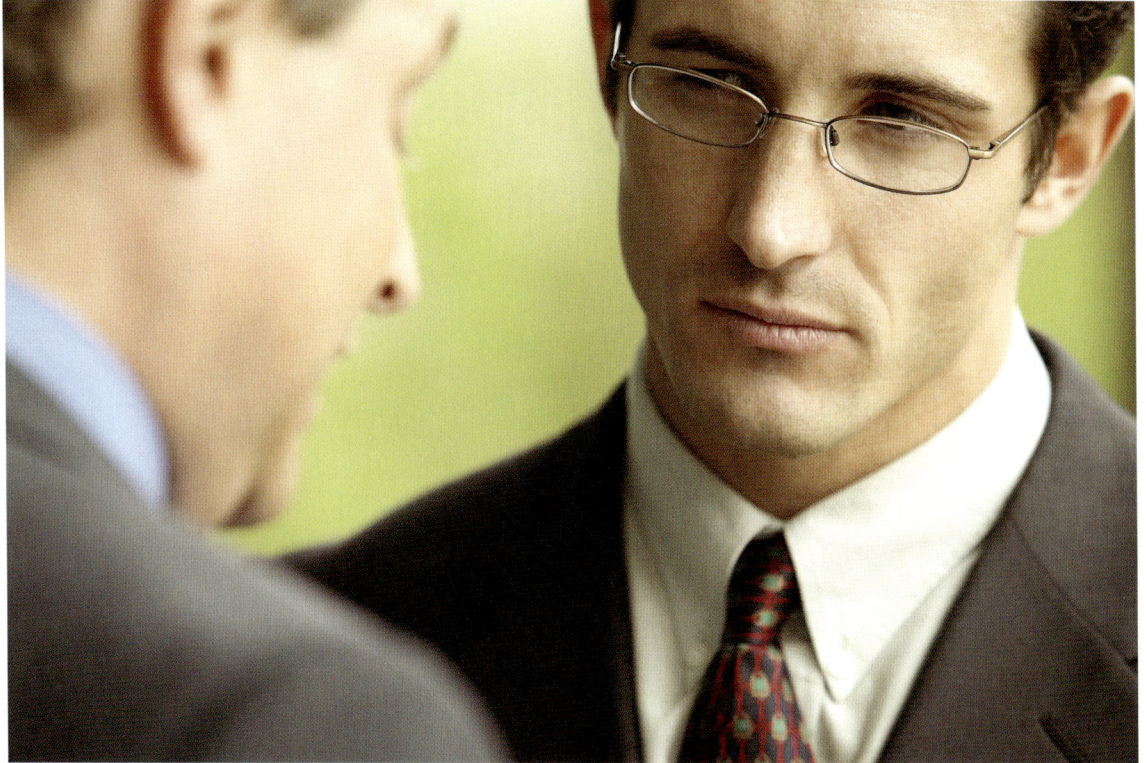
Criminal psychologists interview criminal suspects and witnesses.

The Criminal Psychologist as Police Consultant

Perhaps the role most closely associated with criminal psychology is that of the psychiatrist, psychologist, counselor, therapist, or FBI agent who advises police departments about specific crimes. Television characters like *Law & Order's* Dr. Emil Skoda and *Law & Order: SVU's* Dr. George Huang and movie roles like Clarice Starling in *The Silence of the Lambs* reinforce the idea that criminal psychology focuses solely on predicting criminal behavior. While criminal psychologists *do* assist police departments in under-

Fields That Use
Criminal-Psychology Expertise

law enforcement
criminal justice system
corrections system
treatment settings
counseling
education
ministry
nonprofit work
public awareness and
 crime prevention
technology development
print media (newspapers, magazines, books, etc.)
entertainment industry (movies, TV, etc.)
legislation

standing criminals and how they behave, they also help law enforcement agencies in other ways.

- *They analyze crime scenes.* The choice of crime scene can say something about both the victim and the perpetrator. When a person is killed at home, for example, the home itself can say much about the victim. A spotless, overly tidy home suggests attention to detail, care, perfectionism, organizational tendencies, and perhaps a desire to please people or be in control. To the criminal psychologist it also suggests the person who lived there would not be careless about opening the door to strangers. A criminal psychologist could look at the crime scene to learn about the person who lived in the home, and then determine if the crime was most likely committed by a stranger or someone known to the victim. She might also be asked to make observations about the perpetrator. Was he organized or disorganized? Was he in control and deliberate when he committed the murder, or was this a crime of passion? Crime scenes are not silent witnesses; they hold many clues for the trained eye.

- *They analyze people involved in cases under investigation.* Suppose a man is found dead behind the wheel of a car lying crushed at the bottom of a ravine next to a long stretch of isolated highway. Is it suicide, murder, or accidental death? Did he drive through the guardrail on purpose, did someone tamper with his car, or did he fall asleep at the wheel? The insurance company who carries the deceased's life insurance needs to know; millions of dollars are riding on the answer. A criminal psychologist might be asked to interview the man's friends, family, coworkers, and those who saw him last to help determine if his death was a suicide.

- *They help investigators to more effectively interview criminal suspects and witnesses.* When police investigators interview witnesses and criminal suspects, they don't just ask questions. They've been trained to handle certain people in specific ways. Detectives won't interview a grieving widow with no record who is suspected in her spouse's murder the same way they would interview a known criminal who witnesses identified as shooting the victim. Different interview subjects require different interviewing techniques. Training, however, doesn't cover every type of interviewee or every situation. Detectives might call in a criminal psychologist to help them understand with whom they are dealing and how best to approach the interrogation to get the answers they need.

- *They serve as investigative consultants.* Sometimes criminal psychologists serve as experts to whom authorities can go with questions about a criminal's mindset, the possible reasons or motives behind certain crimes, why she chose specific victims, if and where she might strike again, whether certain crimes are related, and a host of other questions that might arise during a criminal investigation. The criminal psychologist may be brought into the department to meet with those working on the case, or he may just provide brief answers over the telephone. In any case, he serves as an informational resource for the people who investigate crimes and catch criminals.

In addition to helping professionals who solve crimes and enforce laws, criminal psychologists also provide assistance to those who work in the legal system after arrests are made.

The Criminal Psychologist as Lawyer Consultant

Police officers and detectives aren't the only ones who want to understand the criminal mind. Lawyers who prosecute and represent them want to know as much as they can about them, too.

Because criminal psychologists know much about how criminals think and act, they can help lawyers better understand those who have

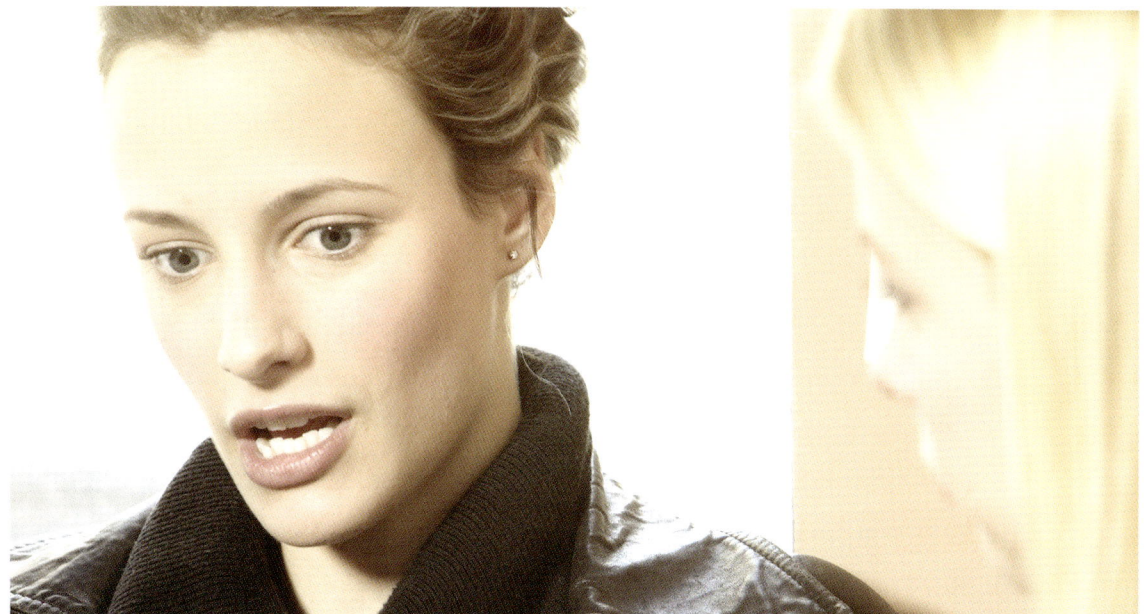

There is no single method of interviewing people. Criminal psychologists must determine which technique works best for the particular individual.

been charged with crimes. Defense attorneys, those who represent the accused criminal in court, use criminal psychologists to help explain why the accused did what she did (if guilty) or why she might have been charged (if innocent). Prosecuting attorneys, those trying to convict the criminal and put her in jail, might consult with criminal psychologists to develop theories or motives for a crime. Before a trial begins, criminal psychologists help lawyers—defense or prosecution—in three primary capacities.

- *They evaluate the accused.* Criminal psychologists can perform standardized personality and intelligence tests on those accused of a crime to help lawyers learn more about them. They can assess the accused for signs of mental illness or psychological disorders. They can also

The Many Roles of a Criminal Psychologist

provide input about whether the accused understands enough of what is happening to him to be tried in a court of law. One key element criminal psychologists look for in evaluating those standing trial is the defendant's mental state at the time of the crime; was he insane or experiencing a mental defect when he committed the act for which he is charged?

- *They assist in preparing witnesses to testify.* Criminal psychologists don't just work with criminals; they help witnesses, too. A prosecuting attorney in a rape case might ask a criminal psychologist to work with a rape victim to help her prepare mentally and emotionally for what she'll go through in court. The same might be done for a battered spouse or an abused child. Criminal psychologists don't ever tell witnesses what to say; they only prepare witnesses for what they will experience during a trial.

- *During the jury-selection process, they offer input as to who would and who would not make the best jurors for their lawyer's side.* Based on basic information that has been provided to them, criminal psychologists can "read" people and make detailed observations about their likely opinions and actions. When dealing with jury selection, lawyers may consult criminal psychologists to identify jurors who would most likely be sympathetic to their side of the courtroom drama. In the United States, lawyers may also use criminal psychologists to help determine whether a prospective juror would be willing to impose the death penalty, should the accused be convicted in a potential death-penalty case.

Once the trial begins, a criminal psychologist can still be used in several ways.

Other Areas of Competency to Which a Criminal Psychologist Might Testify

While criminal psychologists often testify about a person's ability to stand trial, aid in representation, represent himself if he so desires, or testify in court, their expertise at determining competency isn't limited to those areas. A criminal psychologist may also be asked to determine if a person was competent to:

- waive his legal right to be silent
- waive his legal right to have a lawyer present during questioning
- consent to a police search
- consent to a police seizure
- provide and sign a confession
- plead guilty
- refuse counsel
- refuse an insanity defense
- be criminally responsible for the act he committed

The Criminal Psychologist as Court Consultant

A criminal psychologist can be called by the defense or the prosecution, or they can be appointed by the court. In each of these capacities, she can do any of the following.

- *She can evaluate an individual's competency to self-represent, stand trial, or testify.* While lawyers may have already asked a criminal psychologist to perform these duties, a judge can order a defendant or witness to be evaluated as well. In these cases, the court appoints an evaluator (often a psychiatrist or criminal psychologist) to meet with, test, or diagnose the person being evaluated. The evaluator then reports back to the court with her findings.

- *She can evaluate the validity of eyewitness testimony.* When a person witnesses a crime or identifies a suspect in a police lineup, many factors come into play including vision, lighting, visual memory, auditory memory, how open the witness is to suggestion, emotions at the time of the crime, emotions at the time of the identification, self-confidence, and social pressures and expectations. Dynamics occur in these situations that psychologists can help the layperson understand. Criminal psychologists are often called to affirm or cast doubt on eyewitness accounts and identifications by examining these dynamics. They can testify about psychological phenomena that occur during intensely emotional times that might color the witness's ability to give accurate testimony. Take, for example, five people who witness a drunk-driving accident. All five people may give different accounts of what happened. Whose account is most

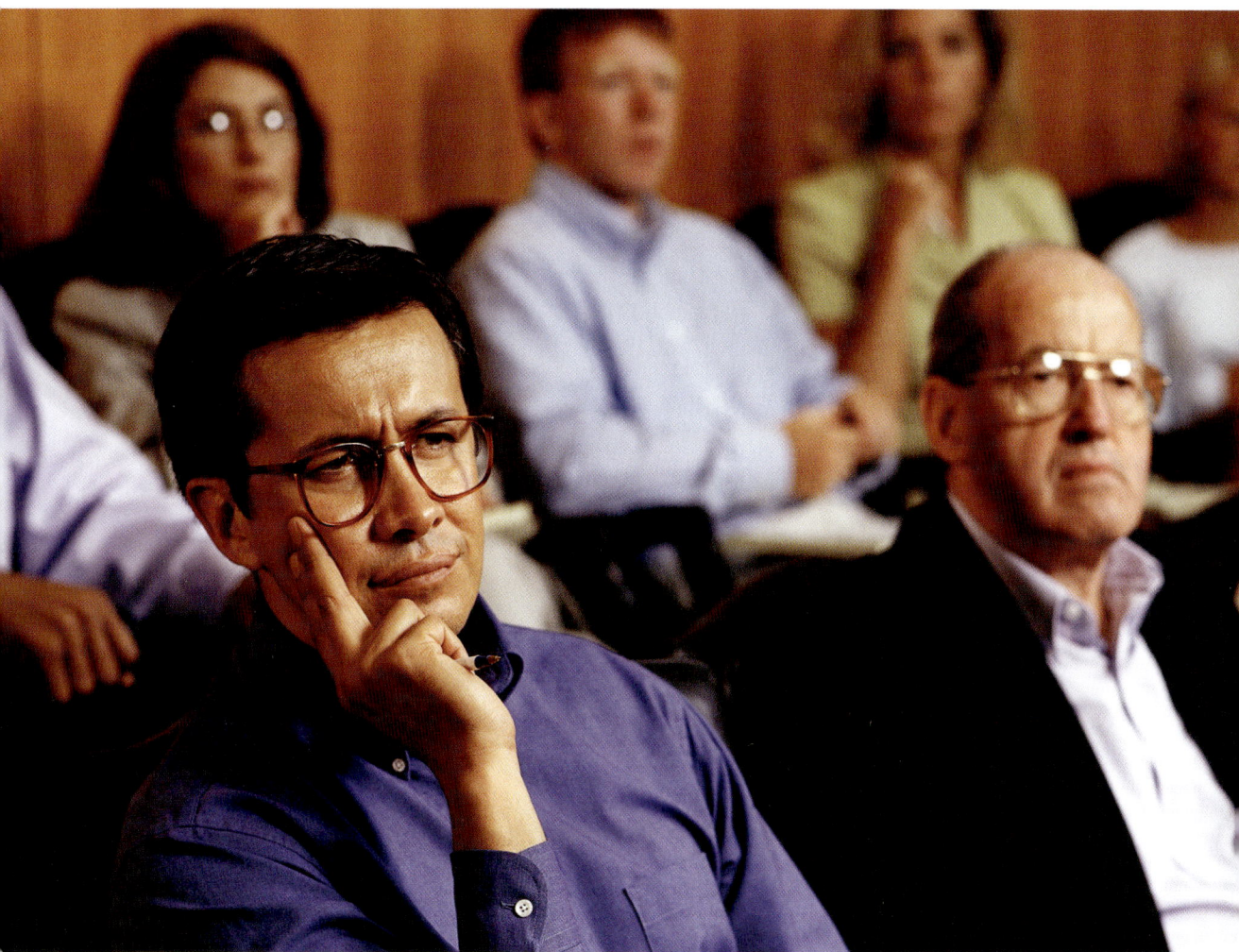

Criminal psychologists often testify in trials. They must present evidence in a way that jurors will be able to understand.

accurate? Which eyewitness is most reliable? What if the driver is a Caucasian male in a Hispanic or other ethnic neighborhood? What if he is a Hispanic male in a Caucasian neighborhood? What social conditions could influence eyewitnesses? Criminal psychologists shed light on these factors.

The Many Roles of a Criminal Psychologist   37

Topics a Criminal Psychologist Might Be Asked to Testify About in Court

- Does the personality of a deceased person suggest anything about how he might have died?
- Is the defendant competent to stand trial (can he understand legal proceedings)?
- Was the defendant sane when he committed the offense?
- Does the defendant know the difference between right and wrong?
- How likely is it that the defendant can be rehabilitated?
- Is the defendant mentally ill or in need of mental-health services?
- How might a defendant's past have influenced his behavior?
- Did the defendant's conduct during the commission of the crime suggest he might repeat the crime if released?
- Is a person involved in a case competent to give testimony?
- What psychological consequences has the crime victim experienced as a result of the crime?
- Does a mentally ill person pose a threat to himself or others?
- How reliable is an eyewitness's testimony?
- What emotional factors could have biased an eyewitness?
- What affect would a delay in trial procedure have on a defendant, the victim, or other witnesses?

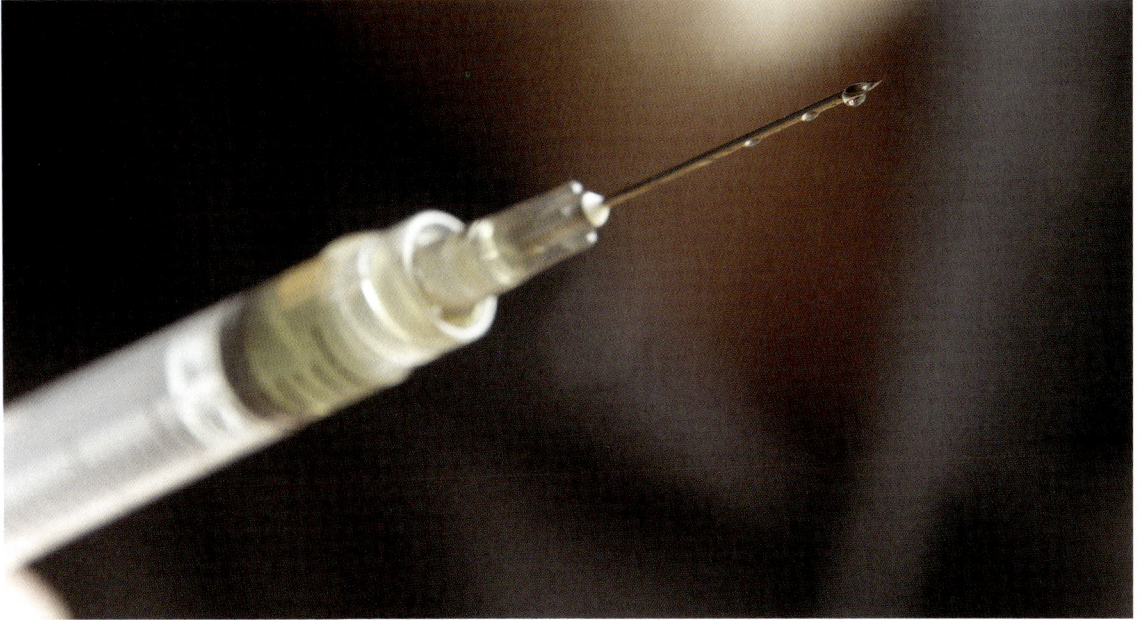

A criminal psychologist determines whether a suspect is mentally competent and therefore a candidate for lethal injection (or some other form of the death penalty).

- *She can evaluate a convicted criminal's competency to receive the death penalty.* Canada abolished the death penalty in its criminal justice system, but in some states in the United States, convicted criminals can be sentenced to die for their crimes. Death sentences can only be given, however, if the convict is deemed competent: that is, if he is capable of understanding what is happening to him and why. In most states the mentally impaired and children under a certain age (usually fifteen or sixteen years) cannot be given the death penalty because courts assume they don't have the reasoning ability to understand the finality of a death sentence and its relationship to their crimes.

The Many Roles of a Criminal Psychologist   **39**

- *She can assess whether mitigating circumstances are sufficient to spare a death-penalty candidate from the death penalty.* When the prosecutor in a case asks for the death penalty, the defense attorney will ask a criminal psychologist to determine if there are any mitigating factors from the criminal's childhood, personality, or mental ability that would lead the jury to sentence the defendant to something

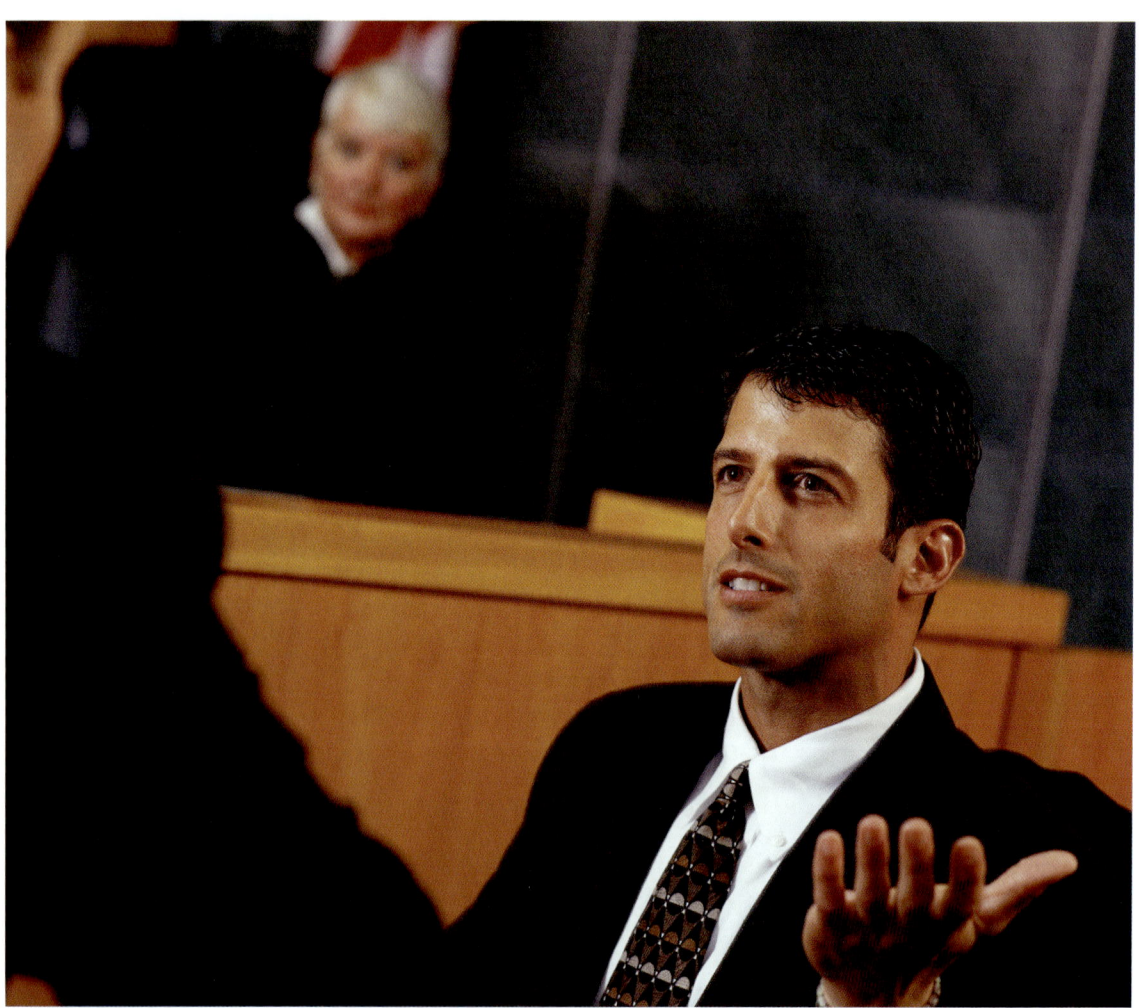

To be an effective expert witness, a criminal psychologist must know about laws and courtroom procedures.

less than death. Mitigating factors are those things that would allow the jury or judge to treat the defendant more mercifully than the law might otherwise allow. Things like having no previous record, a defendant's age (very young or very old), having a limited understanding of the consequences of his actions, mental illness or impairment, abuse or abandonment in the defendant's childhood, extreme emotions, acting under duress or the influence of another, and so on can affect whether a jury views a defendant as deserving of death. The criminal psychologist can assess and give testimony about whether mitigating circumstances exist and, if they do, explain them.

- *She can provide expert testimony.* Because criminal psychology is not an exact science, the criminal psychologist's role as "expert" witness is often contested by opposing lawyers. It can be a difficult position to be in. As forensic psychologist Katherine Ramsland notes in her work *The Criminal Mind*:

Being an expert witness means much more than simply being skilled in some area and being prepared. The courtroom is highly political, defendants may lie, eyewitnesses may be mistaken, and even the most sincere confession may be false. Knowing what can happen in a case and having some awareness of legal precedents on psychological issues will aid experts in achieving their best presentation.

As the author suggests, criminal psychologists who offer expert testimony don't just need to know about psychology and criminals; they need to know about laws, courtroom procedures, admissibility of evidence, how their own testimony will be viewed, and how it might be contested. The best rules of thumb for expert witnesses in any field, as suggested by author and forensic psychology professor Lawrence S. Wrightsman in *Forensic Psychology*, are these: never lie, never fake data or fudge results, never make conclusions first then fit the data to your conclusions, and don't worry about the win-loss record of your court appearances. Following Wrightsman's advice should help expert witnesses maintain integrity, honesty, and *credibility* on the witness stand.

The Criminal Psychologist as Teacher, Trainer, and Public Educator

In addition to the roles already addressed, criminal psychologists can be involved in law enforcement training and public education. With the recent rise in interest in forensics and criminal profiling sparked by the entertainment industry, most colleges now offer at least basic courses in criminal psychology and the science of crime. Some even offer degree programs. Colleges need professors with expertise in criminal psychology and are increasingly recruiting them from the ranks of practicing criminal psychologists instead of from the academic world.

Law enforcement training academies need educators, too. How else will police-academy students or FBI recruits learn about the processes involved in criminal psychology and profiling? Most police forces offer basic training in these areas as well for their existing officers. Criminal psychology and profiling, once sneered at by law enforcement officials as quackery and voodoo investigative techniques, are now embraced as important resources on which investigators can draw in their quest to solve crimes. While criminal psychology and profiling don't solve crimes themselves, both can help detectives do so when used with solid evidence-gathering and assessment skills.

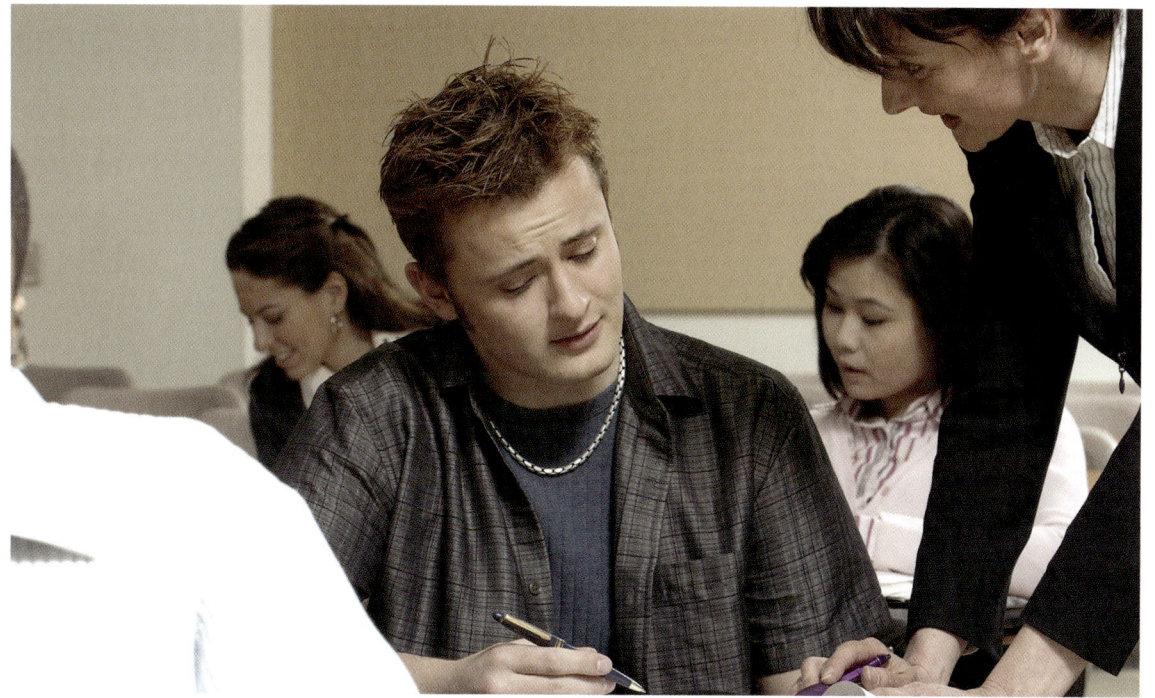

A criminal psychologist may teach her profession at a university or college.

One last, often-overlooked, area in which criminal psychologists can serve is the arena of the public good. They can help people understand crime. Their expertise can help average citizens learn how to avoid becoming crime victims. They can offer insight into how individuals become criminals and what can be done to prevent that from happening. They can help legislators understand what kinds of laws will be most effective in protecting average citizens. They can give domestic violence, abuse, and rape victims the courage to get help.

The person who opts to pursue a career in criminal psychology has many options. Virtually all those options require years of training and education, but perhaps the most difficult career to break into is that of the profiler.

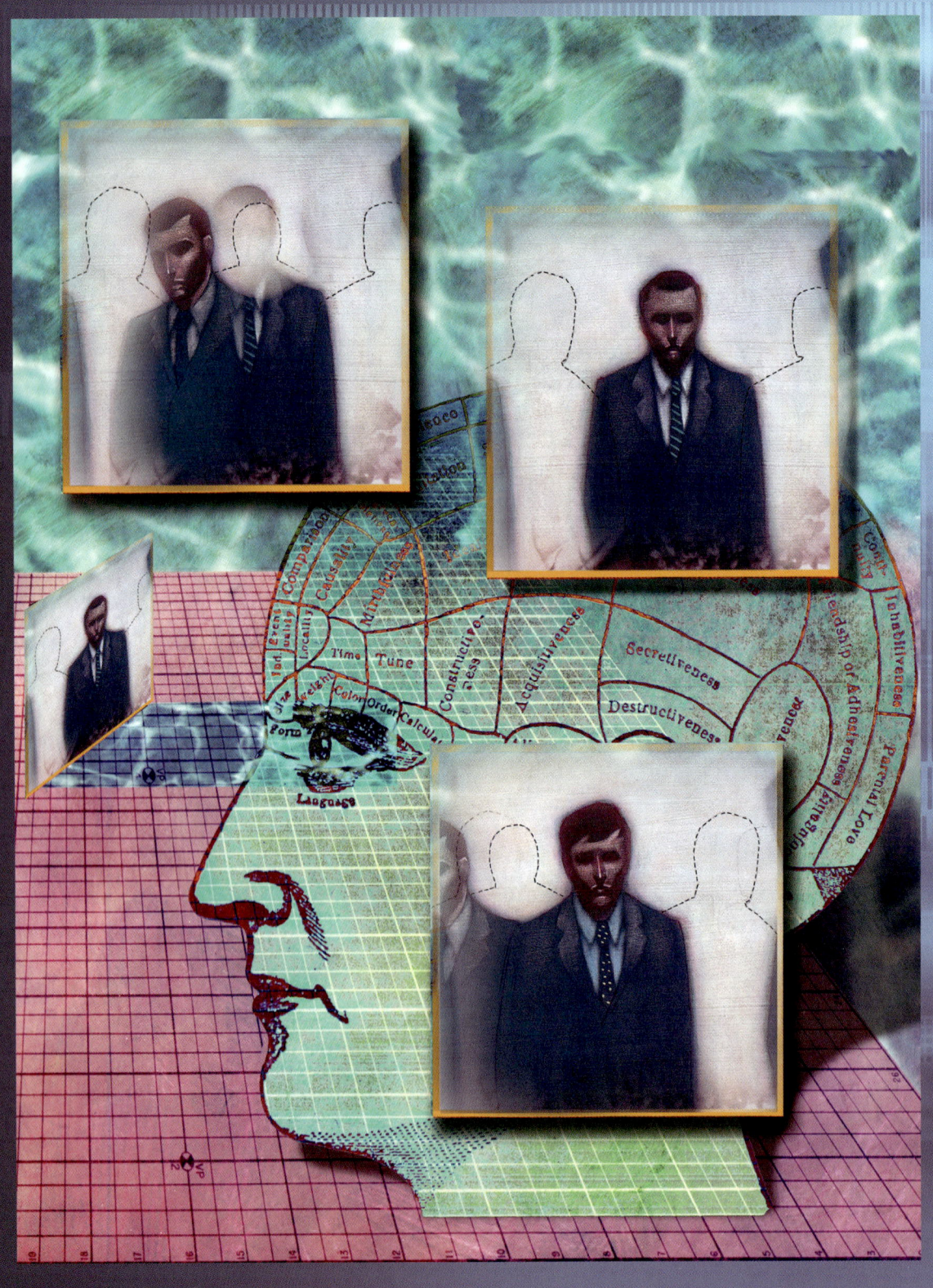

THE PROFILER

From a press release issued in November 2001:

Based on . . . the "weapon" of choice . . . the offender:

- is likely an adult male.
- if employed, is likely to be in a position requiring little contact with the public, or other employees. He may work in a laboratory. He is apparently comfortable working with an extremely hazardous material. He probably has a scientific background to some extent, or at least a strong interest in science.
- has likely taken appropriate protective steps to ensure his own safety, which may include the use of a . . . vaccination or antibiotics.

- has access to a source of [his weapon of choice] and possesses knowledge and expertise to refine it.
- possesses or has access to some laboratory equipment.
- has exhibited an organized, rational thought process in furtherance of his criminal behavior.
- has a familiarity, direct or indirect, with the Trenton, NJ, metropolitan area.
- did not select victims randomly. He made an effort to identify the correct address, including zip code, of each victim and used sufficient postage to ensure proper delivery of the letters. . . . These targets are probably very important to the offender. They may have been the focus of previous expressions of contempt which may have been communicated to others, or observed by others.
- is a nonconfrontational person, at least in his public life. He lacks the personal skills necessary to confront others. He chooses to confront his problems "long distance" and not face-to-face. He may hold grudges for a long time, vowing that he will get even with "them" one day. There are probably other, earlier examples of this type of behavior. . . . He may have chosen to anonymously harass other individuals or entities that he perceived as having wronged him. He may also have chosen to utilize the mail on those occasions.
- prefers being by himself more often than not. If he is involved in a personal relationship, it will likely be of a self-serving nature.

PRE-OFFENSE BEHAVIOR

- Following the events of September 11, 2001, this person may have become mission oriented in his desire to undertake these . . . mailings. He may have become more secretive and exhibited an unusual pattern of activity. Additionally, he may have displayed a passive

CRIMINAL PSYCHOLOGY & PERSONALITY PROFILING

disinterest in the events which otherwise captivated the Nation. He also may have started taking antibiotics unexpectedly.

POST-OFFENSE BEHAVIOR

- He may have exhibited significant behavioral changes at various critical periods of time throughout the course of the . . . mailings and related media coverage. These may include:

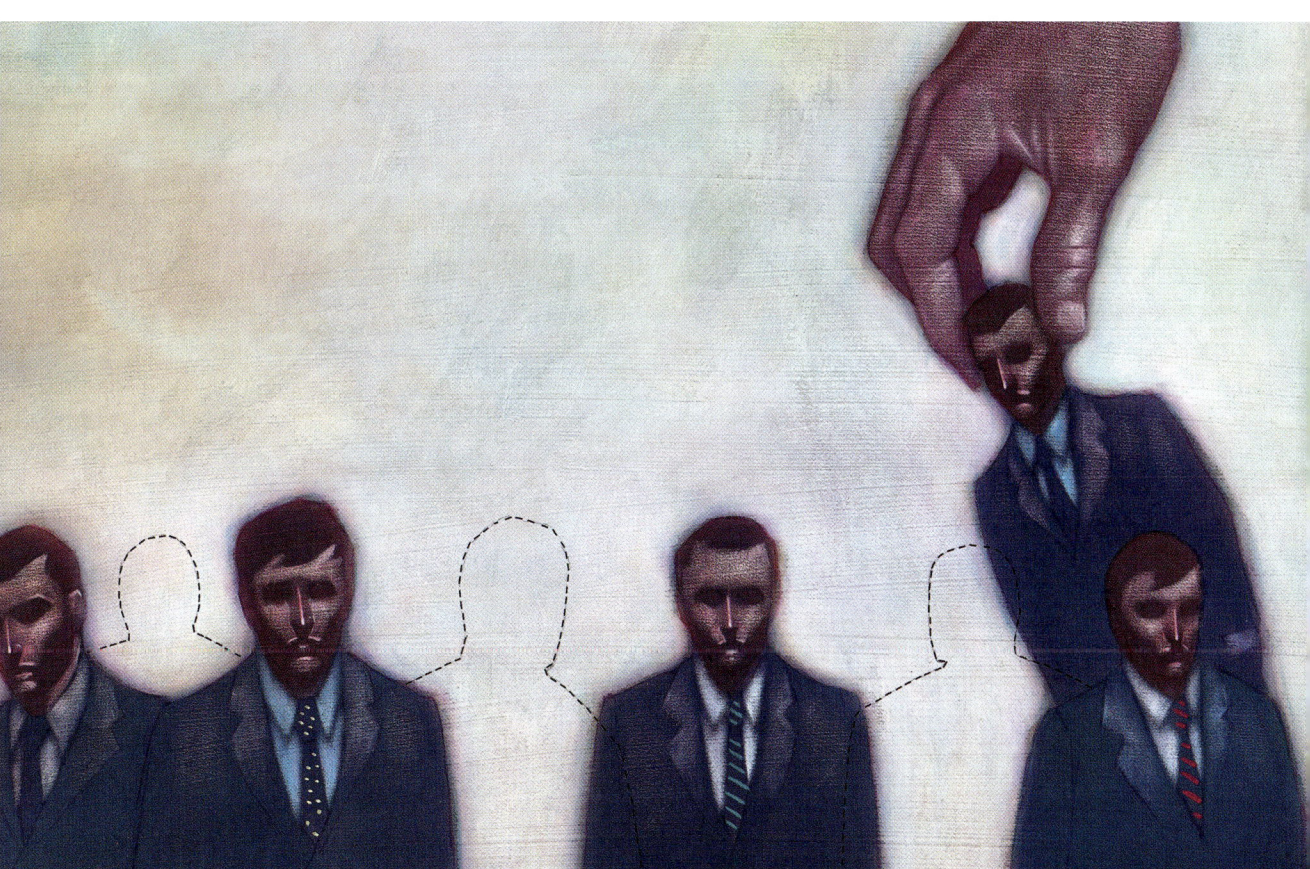

A psychological profile can help investigators narrow down suspects. It is just one of many ways to help solve crimes.

1. Altered physical appearance.
2. Pronounced anxiety.
3. *Atypical* media interest.
4. Noticeable mood swings.
5. More withdrawn.
6. Unusual level of preoccupation.
7. Unusual absenteeism.
8. Altered sleeping and/or eating habits.

These post-offense behaviors would have been most noticeable during critical times, including but not limited to: the mailing of the letters (09/18/01 and 10/09/01), the death of [the] first . . . victim, media reports of each . . . incident, and especially the deaths and illnesses of non-targeted victims.

These lists and paragraphs are part of an actual behavioral assessment included in an FBI press briefing given in November 2001. At the time of this press release, the FBI was seeking help in identifying the person who sent seven anthrax-laced letters through the mail to five news agencies and two senatorial offices, killing five people and infecting seventeen more.

Anthrax, an infectious disease caused by spore-forming bacteria that affects animal and human skin, lungs, or intestines, can be fatal if inhaled. The U.S. Centers for Disease Control and Prevention (CDC) classifies anthrax as a Category A priority substance with recognized bioterrorism potential. According to the CDC, Category A agents are those that:

- pose the greatest possible threat for a bad effect on public health
- may spread across a large area or need public awareness
- need a great deal of planning to protect the public's health

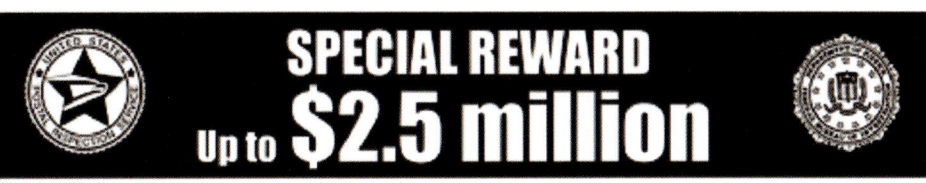

SPECIAL REWARD
Up to $2.5 million

For information leading to the arrest and conviction of the individual(s) responsible for the mailing of letters containing anthrax to the New York Post, Tom Brokaw at NBC, Senator Tom Daschle and Senator Patrick Leahy:

**AS A RESULT OF EXPOSURE TO ANTHRAX,
FIVE (5) PEOPLE HAVE DIED.**

The person responsible for these deaths...

- Likely has a scientific background/work history which may include a specific familiarity with anthrax
- Has a level of comfort in and around the Trenton, NJ area due to present or prior association

Anyone having information, contact **America's Most Wanted** at **1-800-CRIME TV** or the **FBI** via e-mail at **amerithrax@fbi.gov**

All information will be held in strict confidence. Reward payment will be made in accordance with the conditions of Postal Service Reward Poster 296, dated February 2000. Source of reward funds: U.S. Postal Service and FBI $2,000,000; ADVO, Inc. $500,000.

Press release from November 2001

Again according to the CDC, most cases of anthrax limited to the skin can be cured if treated early with antibiotics. Even if untreated, 80 percent of those who become infected with skin anthrax do not die. Gastrointestinal anthrax, the kind you get if you ingest anthrax, is more serious: between one-fourth and more than half of these cases lead to death. Inhalation anthrax, the kind you get in your lungs—the kind the killer sent in the mail in 2001—is much more severe: more than 50 percent of people with inhalation anthrax die.

The person who mailed the letters deliberately inserted anthrax spores into envelopes so that whoever opened the letters would inhale the spores. People in the United States were under biological attack.

The anthrax attacks began just one week after the September 11, 2001, terrorist attack on the Twin Towers in New York City. The first set of letters bore postmarks dated September 18, 2001; the second batch, which contained a more potent type of anthrax, were postmarked October 9, 2001. Both were mailed from Trenton, New Jersey.

The U.S. government and its people, nervous from the unprecedented targeting of innocent civilians on North American shores, expected more attacks. Law enforcement officials and the public felt tense and restless. Americans wanted the terror to end. The FBI needed to find the person behind these letters before public panic erupted. But investigative agencies had little evidence to go on: no fingerprints, no DNA, no witnesses, no suspects. It would take weeks to identify the specific anthrax strains and grades used in the letters, the sources of the anthrax spores, and the people who had greatest access to these strains. But the directors of the agencies involved felt that to save lives they needed to move quickly. They developed a profile of the offender.

The letters provided clues about who wrote them. The points of origin; the choice of poison contained in each one; the letters' content, writing

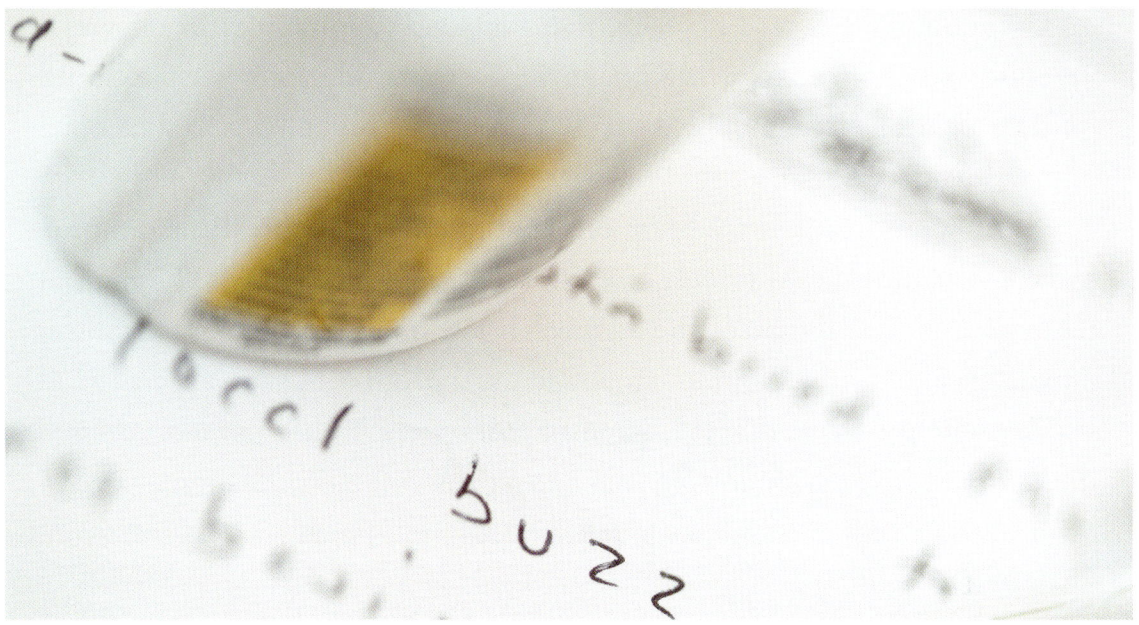

A criminal's handwriting may contain clues about his personality.

styles, and handwriting itself, all provided information with which criminal psychologists could develop a list of traits thought to be true of the unknown offender. That's all a profile is—a list of characteristics—based on certain theories, facts, and evidence—that summarize the offender's probable background and personality. Once the FBI's behavioral scientists came up with their profile of the anthrax mail terrorist, they asked "the American public to study these assessments and reflect on whether someone of their acquaintance might fit the profile." When it released its profile, the agency stated "the safety of the American people is at stake."

News agencies, national media, television programs, and magazines carried the profile. It made front-page news. The FBI circulated reward posters containing key parts of the profile. The same reward posters showed up in local post offices all over the United States. Reproductions of the profile in full appeared in local and regional newspapers.

Despite the FBI's plea for help, their detailed linguistic and behavioral profiles, and their offer of a $2.5 million reward, the case wasn't closed until 2010. The FBI eventually focused on biologist Bruce Ivins, but he committed suicide before he could be charged.

In the anthrax case, a team of experts from the Critical Incident Response Group of the National Center for the Analysis of Violent Crime put together the description of the suspect listed on the FBI's reward poster and in the behavioral profile contained in the press release excerpted at the beginning of this chapter. Some of these were highly trained criminal investigators and psychologists who specialize in the personality and character traits of people who have committed crimes. We call these professionals criminal profilers.

The Criminal Profiler

The term "profiler" generally refers to someone who studies the known traits, records, and tendencies of a person or entity. The profiler summarizes that information into a report, the profile. Think of a drawing done in profile—the image captures only the outline of the side of the head; it isn't a complete, detailed drawing. It's a visual summary. A profiler's profile is a summary, too, but it uses words. Profilers and profiles can be found in many professions.

A corporation may use an economist to develop a financial profile that provides concise information about the company's net worth—a summary of the company's financial status. An employer may ask job applicants to take personality tests to develop profiles about their potential suitability for a job—summaries of their strengths and weaknesses. Handwriting experts may be asked to examine written letters or historical documents to confirm authorship or to develop *linguistic* profiles of the writers—summaries of the

Key Murder Elements for Profilers

- killing site: where the murder took place
- disposal site: where the body was found
- position of the body (degrading position indicates loathing)
- presence of head coverings or blindfolds (depersonalizes the victim)
- indications of bondage (suggests planning and organization)
- use of duct tape (indicates perpetrator spent time in prison)
- facial wounds (depersonalizes the victim)
- weapon used
- evidence of staging (the criminal altered the crime scene)
- souvenirs taken by the perpetrator (a reminder of the crime, often an object that belonged to the victim)
- trophies taken by the perpetrator (a reminder of the crime and a visual reward that arouses the killer)

writers' skills, understanding, and specific use of words. Psychologists or psychiatrists may work as psychological profilers, making generalizations about the people they examine based on interviews with the persons involved, their histories, and their known behaviors—summaries of personalities and people types. Again, these are brief, condensed character sketches of complex individuals. They are word summaries, or profiles, of their subjects.

The criminal profiler, as the term implies, develops summaries about people who commit crimes. Because the perpetrator isn't known, the criminal profiler's information comes from crime scenes and victims. According to John Douglas, former chief of the Investigative Support Unit of the FBI's National Center for the Analysis of Violent Crime, the profiler follows several steps in completing the profile process:

- He evaluates the criminal act itself.
- He evaluates the specifics of the crime scene or scenes.
- He analyzes the victim or victims.
- He examines preliminary police reports about the crime.
- He evaluates autopsy reports and the medical examiner's methods.
- After completing the above, he develops a profile complete with offender traits.
- Finally, he makes suggestions to investigators based on his research and profile.

None of the above would do any good, however, if the following statement weren't true: Criminals say much about themselves in their crimes. In fact, this truth provides the foundation from which profilers work. How criminals reveal themselves in their crimes is further defined in four assumptions made by every criminal profiler.

Four Assumptions of the Profiler

1. *Crimes scenes reflect their criminals' personalities.* In other words, what a person does reveals something of who she is.
2. *A criminal will tend to use the same or similar modus operandi—method of operation (MO)—in each crime.* An MO consists of actions the criminal takes that are necessary to complete the crime (using a nylon cord to

Traits of Organized, Disorganized, and Mixed Offenders:

organized:
- average to above-average intelligence
- socially competent
- most likely skilled
- sexually capable
- birth order: first or second born
- father had stable job
- inconsistent childhood discipline
- controlled emotions during crime
- alcohol used during crime
- lives with a partner
- drives to crime scene in well-maintained car
- shows interest in media attention
- learns from each crime, hones skill

disorganized:
- below-average intelligence
- socially inadequate
- usually unskilled
- sexually incapable
- birth order: youngest
- father's work unstable
- harsh childhood punishment
- anxious during crime
- minimal or no use of alcohol
- lives alone
- works/lives near crime scene
- has little interest in media
- stays disorganized

Mixed offenders display traits from both columns.

strangle a victim, wearing gloves to avoid leaving fingerprints, cutting the victim's telephone and electric lines before breaking in, etc.).

3. *A criminal's "signature" remains the same.* A signature differs from an MO. While the MO includes what was necessary for the crime, the signature covers actions taken during the crime that are unnecessary for the successful completion of the crime, that are unique to that criminal, and that satisfy the criminal's emotional needs. Signatures might include things like certain words the offender utters while committing the crime (for example, a serial rapist muttering "whore" while raping his victim), leaving certain items in specific places at the crime scene (for instance, resting victims' driver's licenses on their dead bodies), posing the bodies in specific positions, using certain distinguishing techniques (surgical incisions instead of careless stab wounds), or leaving markings, notes, or writings on the victims or at the crime scene (for example, leaving a note saying "I will kill again").

4. *The criminal's personality will not change.* Even though we can alter certain behaviors and attitudes (we can quit smoking, or stop swearing, or try to be more patient, for example), we can't change the core of who we are. The same holds true for criminals. And that consistency will show up in their crimes.

By assuming criminals reveal themselves in their crimes via these four truths, the criminal profiler can then study crime scenes, MOs, signatures, victims, and other details about specific crimes to make generalizations about—to create a profile of—the unknown subject, the UNSUB, who committed the act(s).

One tool that helps criminal profilers create these profiles is the FBI's classification system for offenders, detailed in the *Crime Classification Manual.* Among other details and crime classifications, this resource classifies perpetrators as "organized," "disorganized," or a mixture of the two.

A Sampling of Facts and What They Might Imply

FACT SET #1: In interviews, friends, family, and coworkers describe a young murder victim as quiet, submissive, and compliant. Yet her body and the crime scene show evidence of prolonged torture.

IMPLICATIONS: Because the victim probably would have done whatever the murderer asked, the murderer tortured her for his own enjoyment.

FACT SET #2: A woman's body is found on the side of a road along a remote, isolated stretch of highway—the only remote section of this road for miles.

IMPLICATIONS: The killer had access to a car or other vehicle, knew how to drive, was strong enough to lift a body in and out of a car, and was familiar with the area in which the body was dumped.

FACT SET #3: A man dies from thirty-seven stab wounds. The crime scene is sloppy, and no attempt was made to hide evidence.

IMPLICATIONS: Because the killer used more force than necessary, he probably knew and was angry with the victim. His act was fueled by rage. Because the crime scene was sloppy, the killing was probably not planned, but rather done in the heat of the moment.

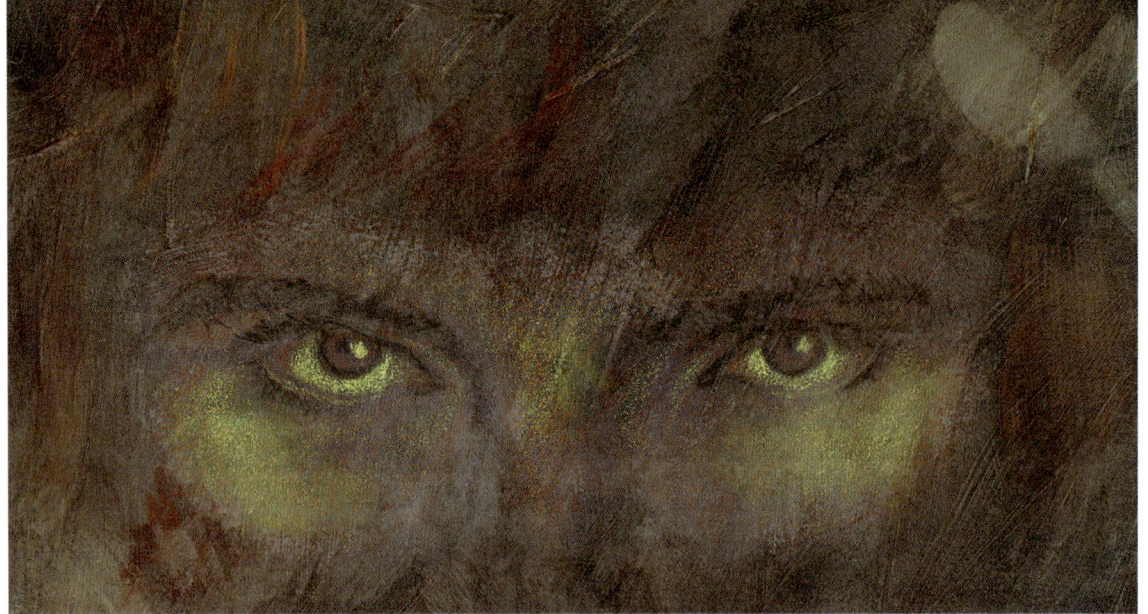

Criminals who are organized can be especially difficult to catch. They carefully plot their crimes and anticipate the moves of law enforcement.

Classifying Perpetrators

Organized offenders commit planned crimes, usually against strangers. The planning is part of the detailed fantasy they've created in their minds. This type of offender selects victims carefully to match what they've imagined. They also want to be certain their victims won't resist them or later identify them. These criminals are calculating, calm, and efficient when they commit their crimes.

Disorganized offenders are careless and impulsive. They're often nervous or anxious when they commit their crimes. They may have to use violence to obtain their victims instead of charm to get them into their grasps. They may commit a crime not because they planned to but simply because the opportunity presented itself. Or they may commit a more serious crime than they intended (murder, for example, in addition to rape) because they lost control of their emotions and actions while committing the initial crime.

Regardless of the criminal or crime involved, each crime scene suggests much about its offender. Where the crime is committed, where a body is left, how the body is left, the way the crime was committed—these suggest organized or disorganized personalities. Once the profiler identifies the UNSUB as organized, disorganized, or mixed, she can predict his behavior in subsequent crimes, sometimes with uncanny accuracy.

In his book *Journey into Darkness*, former FBI profiler John Douglas describes how analyzing a crime scene provides information about a perpetrator, in this case, a child killer:

> Where you find the body, and how quickly you find it, tell us a lot about the killer. Organized killers tend to transport the victims (alive and dead) over distance. They dispose of bodies in places that take longer to find and where conditions may help destroy evidence—in water, for example. Or, they go for drama or shock value, placing the body where it will be found, in a place or condition that will create outrage in the community. As with organized perpetrators of other types of crime, these guys are of average or above-average intelligence and do have social skills. They plan their crimes, targeting strangers indiscriminately . . . , and kill to avoid detection, for the thrill, to fulfill sadistic urges, or for other reasons. Organized child killers may well be psychopathic serial killers. They are more aggressive in sexual activity with their victims before they kill them. Disorganized offenders are more inadequate sexually and so are more likely to assault the victim after the child is unconscious or dead. Of lower intelligence, they frequently don't plan the abduction and often kill

inadvertently. . . . Socially inadequate, they tend to choose a victim they know. Rather than transporting the victim, they feel most comfortable abducting and killing close to home. They may not even have a means to transport a body. Their victims are usually left at the crime scene or someplace where they are found more quickly. They will just dump the body somewhere or bury it in a shallow grave.

A criminal's specific actions indicate definitive traits that are far too numerous to list here. But profilers study these behaviors and the

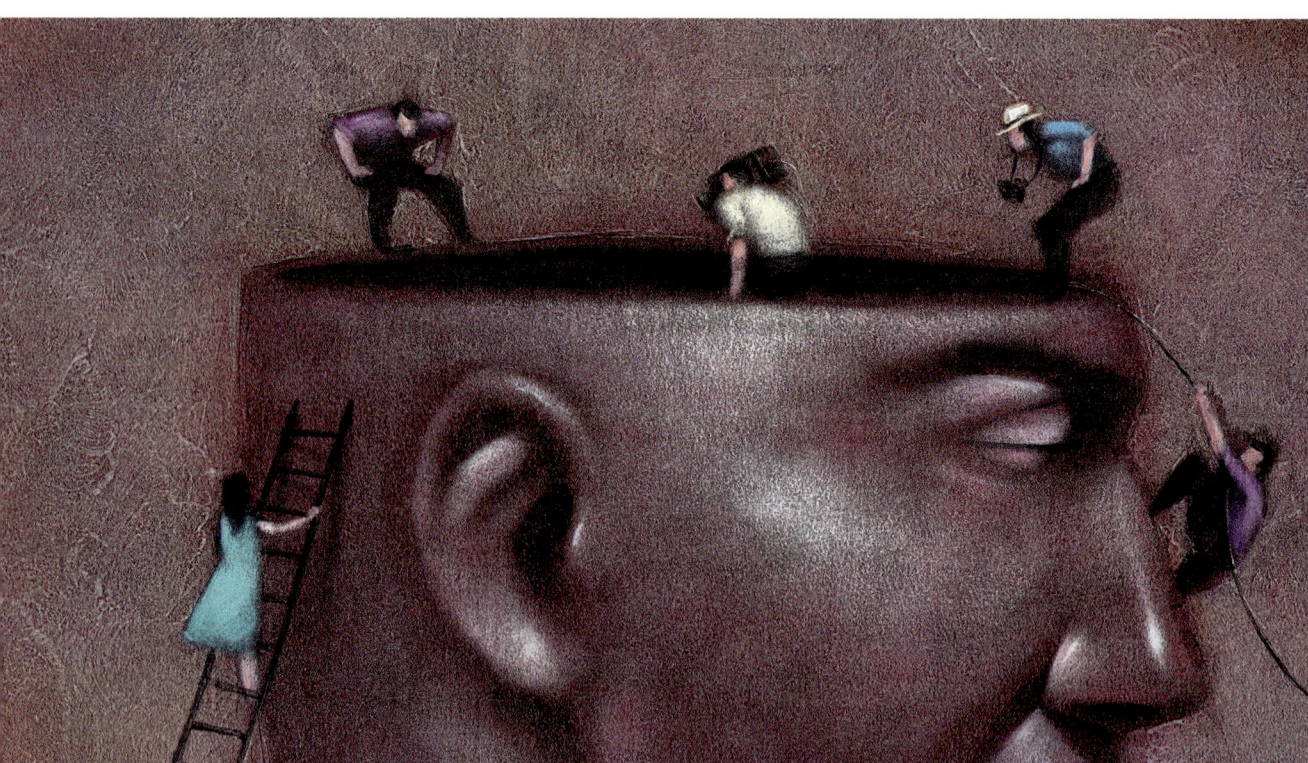

Criminal psychologists study how the offender thinks and behaves.

personalities behind them so much that they are able to "get into" the UNSUB's mind—they learn to think like the perpetrators and to understand their motives. They fill their minds with crime-scene details and **facets** of each crime. They imagine, based on factual evidence, how the crime occurred and what the perpetrator felt. They get into the heads and emotions of the victims, too. And all this comes together in a criminal profile, which investigators use to identify possible suspects and ultimately to capture the criminal responsible for the crime(s).

As you can imagine, criminal profiling can be a dark and ugly business: studying bloody crime-scene photos; listening to cassette tapes of **sadists** torturing their victims; examining horrific, detailed eyewitness descriptions of what victims endured; and hearing the sounds of victims crying and screaming. Criminal profilers have to see and listen to these things; they study them for clues about the perpetrators. And because they do, profilers see humankind's capacity for evil. They live with shocking, horrific images every day. These hardworking men and women see the worst of the worst criminals out there.

As Jim Wright, an investigator with the FBI's Behavioral Science Unit (BSU), put it, "it almost defies description what one person can do to another. . . . There's no way you can be involved in the type of work we're doing or be involved as a law enforcement officer or in the investigation of violent crime and not be personally affected."

But profilers learn to handle it all the same. Part of the ability to handle the darkest parts of the job comes from the individual's strength of character. Part of it comes from being able to divorce job realities from everyday home life. And part of it involves training.

Becoming a Profiler

The process of becoming a profiler isn't easy, particularly one who works for the FBI. Former agent John Douglas describes the process, which is summarized here. First you have to be accepted into the FBI itself. Once you make it through FBI training, you have to demonstrate that you're a solid, top-notch investigator in whatever capacity you're assigned. If you show creativity in your assigned position, the FBI's BSU may recruit you. If they recruit you, and the unit does not select many, you'll be sent to the FBI training center in Quantico, Virginia, where you must pass two additional years of intensive training. Only then will you be admitted into the BSU.

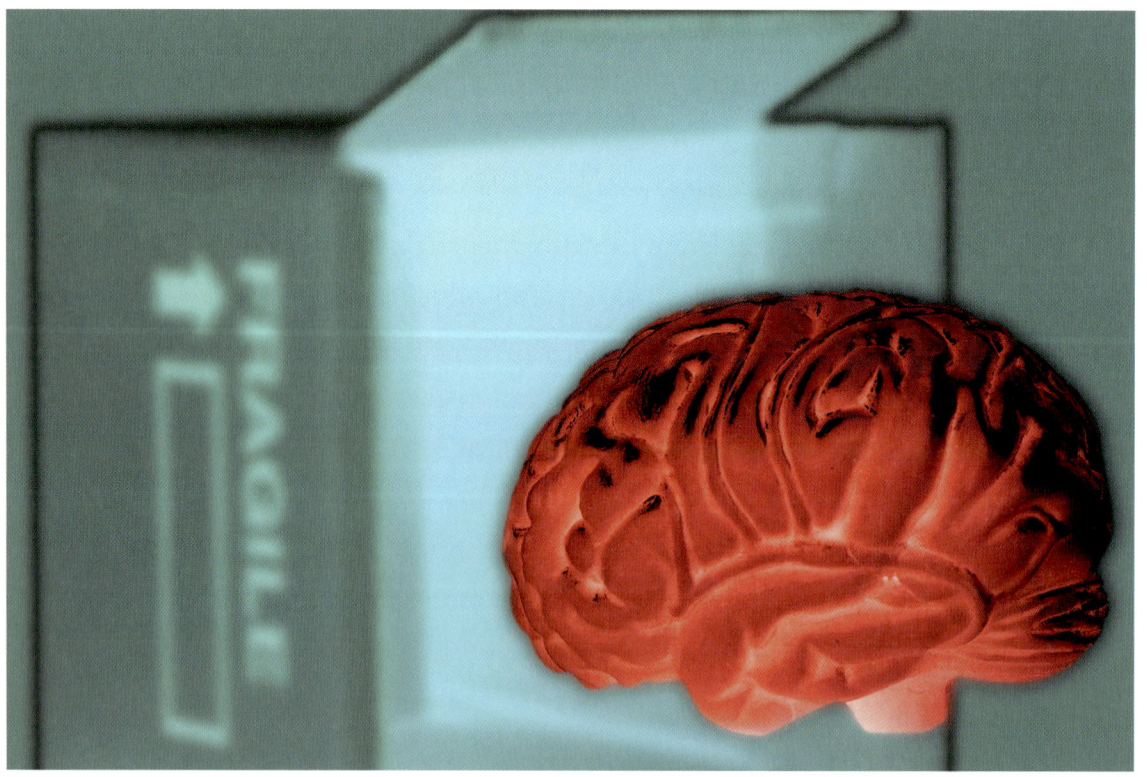

Profilers selected to join the FBI must "think outside the box."

Simply becoming a member of the BSU does not automatically qualify you for a profiling assignment, however. Profilers are hand selected.

Beyond excellent completion of FBI training, senior profilers look for certain characteristics in upcoming professionals. Most hold graduate degrees in their fields, usually doctoral degrees. Good candidates must also, according to Douglas, "show imagination and creativity in investigation." They need to be capable of following rules and **protocols**, but must also be willing to "think outside the box" and take risks. A potential profiler should demonstrate leadership and initiative, but must also be able to work alone or as a member of a team. And, perhaps more than anything else, the potential profiler has to show good judgment: a judgment not only based on fact, but sometimes, according to Douglas, based primarily on instinct. Profiling requires an indefinable talent, a sense or instinct beyond knowledge, that BSU supervisors find hard to explain but are able to identify in candidates.

Becoming a profiler for the FBI sounds glamorous and exciting. The work is rewarding, especially when your profile leads to the arrest and conviction of a criminal. Other times it's frustrating, as in the case of the anthrax terrorist, which took nine years to solve. Most profilers will tell you that criminal profiling is demanding, physically and mentally exhausting, emotionally draining, heartbreaking work—yes, it has its rewards, but it's not the adrenaline-pumping, extrasensory thrill ride portrayed in fiction. In addition to examining crime-scene photos, the profiler's work can involve painstaking research, volumes of reading, and stacks of tedious paperwork. Those who become criminal profilers learn quickly that the job they imagined is far different from reality. Profiling is not what we see on TV.

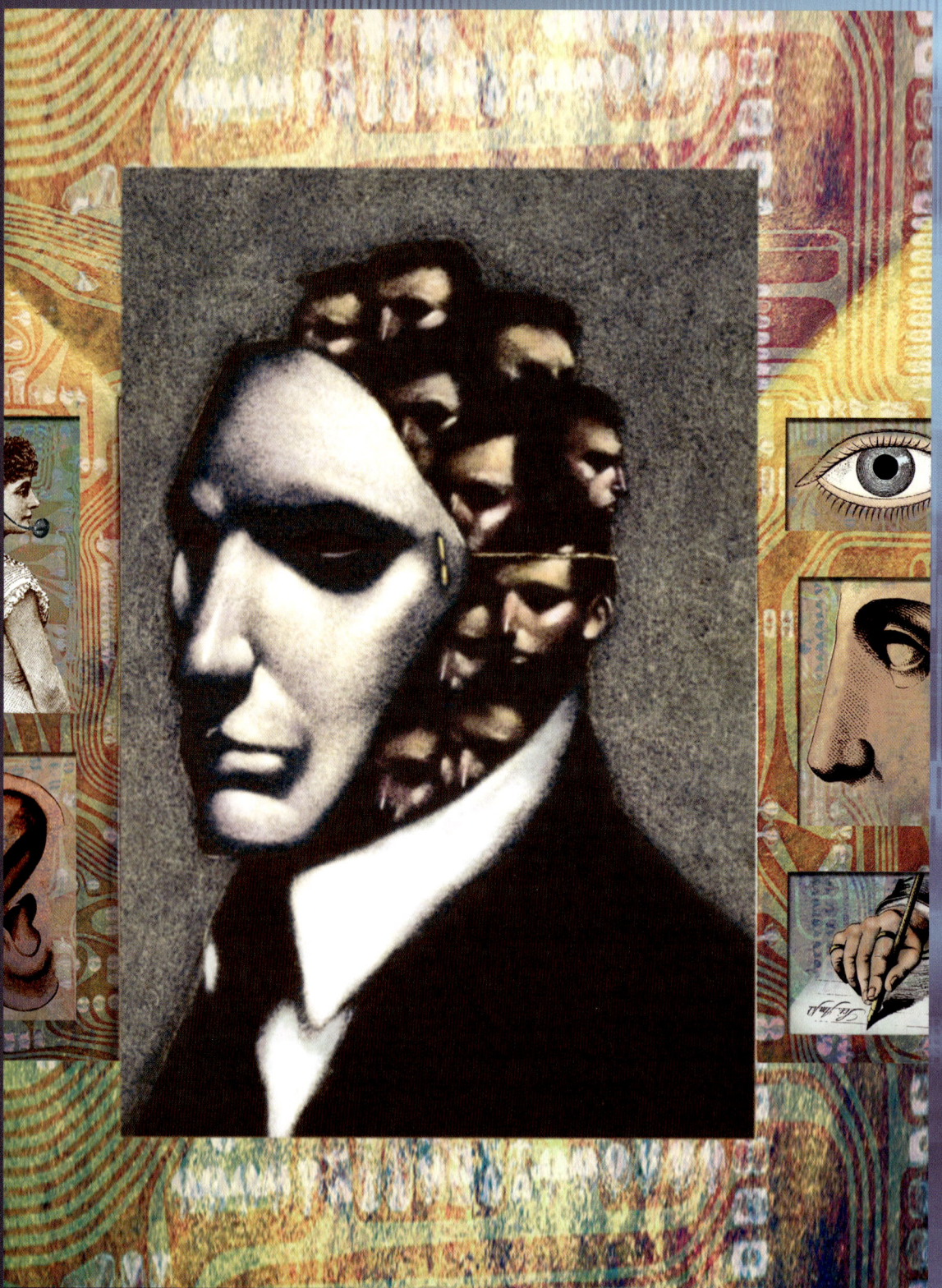

4

CRIMINAL PRO-FILING IN FICTION AND HISTORY

"I have heard you say it is difficult for a man to have any object in daily use without leaving the impress of his individuality upon it in such a way that a trained observer might read it. Now, I have here a watch which has recently come into my possession. Would you have the kindness to let me have an opinion upon the character or habits of the late owner?"

I handed him over the watch with some slight feeling of amusement in my heart, for the test was, as I thought, an impossible one, and I intended it as a lesson against the somewhat dogmatic tone which he occasionally assumed. He balanced the watch in his hand, gazed hard at the dial, opened the back, and examined the works, first with his naked eyes and then with a powerful convex lens. I could hardly keep from smiling at his crestfallen face when he finally snapped the case . . . and handed it back.

"There are hardly any data," he remarked. "The watch has been recently cleaned, which robs me of my most suggestive facts."

"You are right," I answered. "It was cleaned before being sent to me." In my heart I accused my companion of putting forward a most lame and impotent excuse to cover his failure. What data could he expect from an uncleaned watch?

"Though unsatisfactory, my research has not been entirely barren," he observed, staring up at the ceiling with dreamy, lack-lustre eyes. "Subject to your correction, I should judge that the watch belonged to your elder brother, who inherited it from your father."

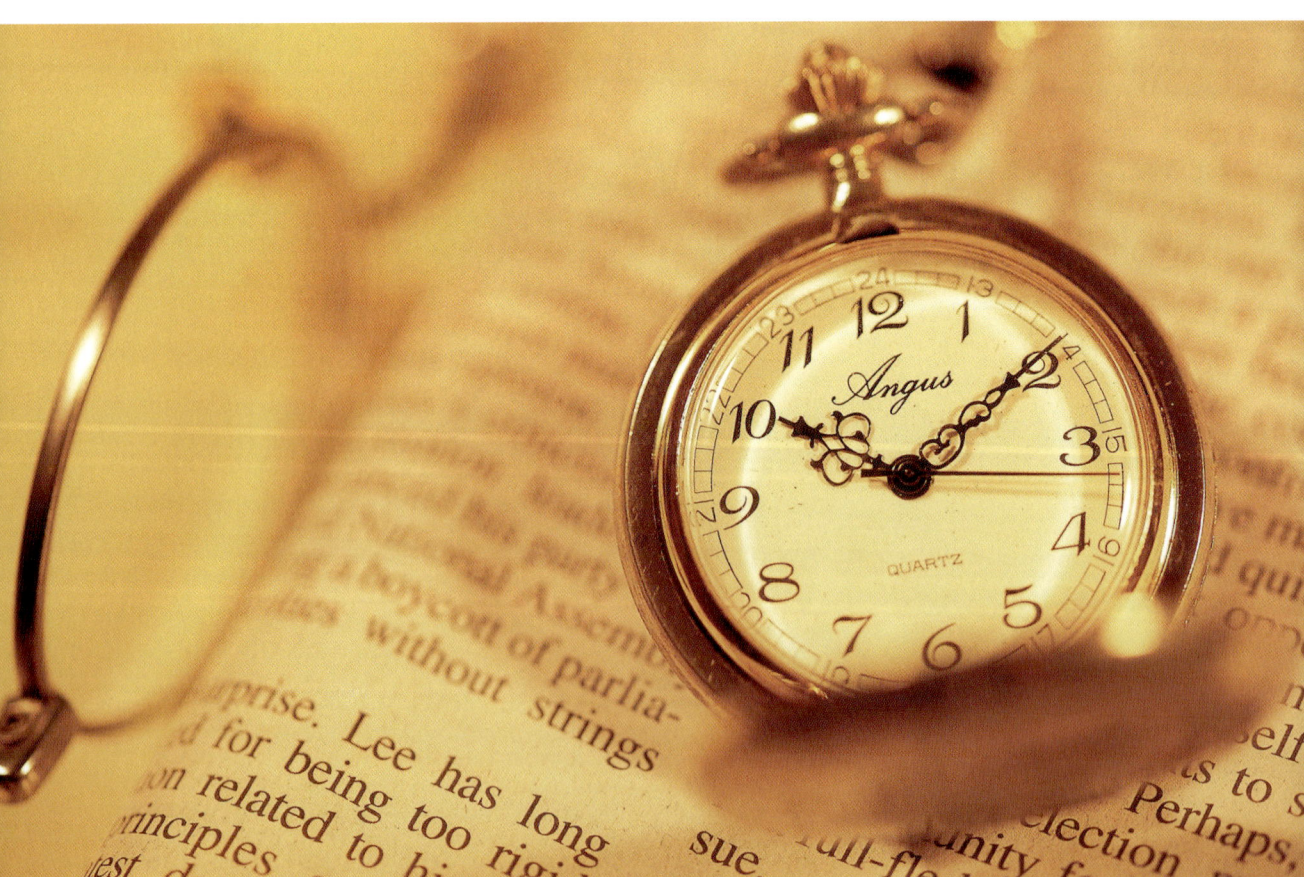

From the ordinary, Sherlock Holmes deduced the extraordinary.

Fast Fact:

French criminologist Dr. Edmond Locard, one of the founders of modern forensic science, was so impressed with the deductive reasoning skills Doyle's character Sherlock Holmes used in his fictional investigations that he recommended that those seeking to become detectives, in addition to their training, study Doyle's works.

"That you gather, no doubt, from the H. W. upon the back?"

"Quite so. The W. suggests your own name. The date of the watch is nearly fifty years back, and the initials are as old as the watch: so it was made for the last generation. Jewelry usually descends to the eldest son, and he is most likely to have the same name as the father. Your father has, if I remember right, been dead many years. It has, therefore, been in the hands of your eldest brother."

"Right, so far," said I. "Anything else?"

"He was a man of untidy habits—very untidy and careless. He was left with good prospects, but he threw away his chances, lived for some time in poverty with occasional short intervals of prosperity, and finally, taking to drink, he died. That is all I can gather."

I sprang from my chair and limped impatiently about the room with considerable bitterness in my heart.

"This is unworthy of you, Holmes," I said. "I could not have believed that you would have descended to this. You have made inquiries into the history of my unhappy brother, and you now pretend to deduce this knowl-

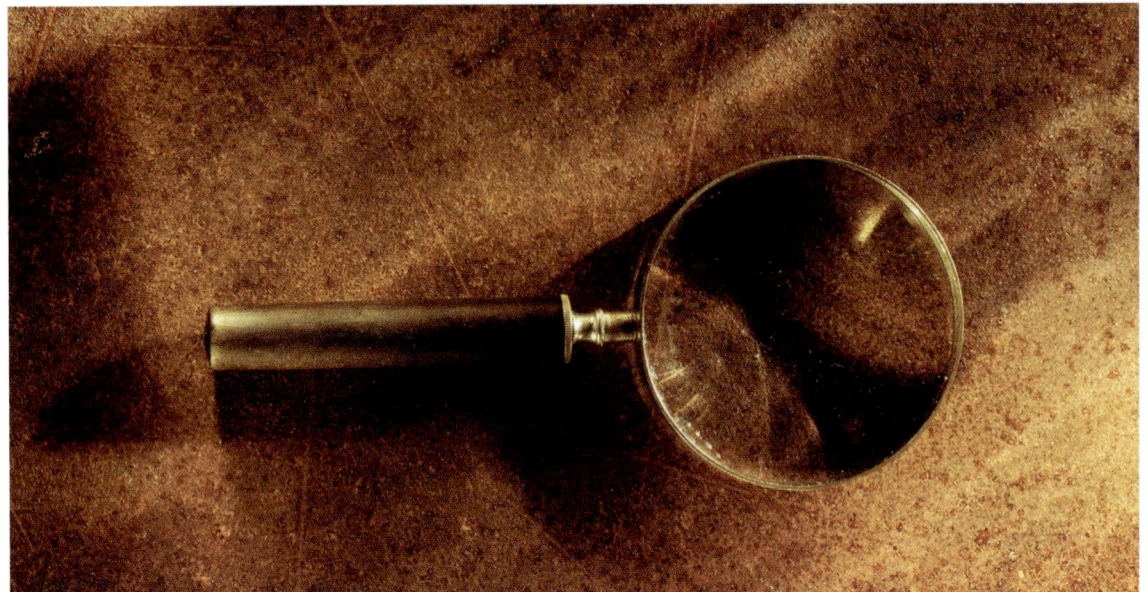

The fictional Sherlock Holmes used his mind and such low-tech tools as a magnifying glass to solve crimes from his home on Baker Street.

edge in some fanciful way. You cannot expect me to believe that you have read all this from his old watch! It is unkind and, to speak plainly, has a touch of **charlatanism** in it."

"My dear doctor," said he kindly, "pray accept my apologies. Viewing the matter as an abstract problem, I had forgotten how personal and painful a thing it might be to you. I assure you, however, that I never even knew that you had a brother until you handed me the watch."

"Then how in the name of all that is wonderful did you get these facts? They are absolutely correct in every particular."

"Ah, that is good luck. I could only say what was the balance of probability. I did not at all expect to be so accurate."

"But it was not mere guesswork?"

"No, no: I never guess. It is a shocking habit—destructive to the logical faculty. What seems strange to you is only so because you do not follow my train of thought or observe the small facts upon which large *inferences* may depend. For example, I began by stating that your brother was careless. When you observe the lower part of that watch-case you notice that it is not only dinted in two places but it is cut and marked all over from the habit of keeping other hard objects, such as coins or keys, in the same pocket. Surely it is no great feat to assume that a man who treats a fifty-guinea watch so *cavalierly* must be a careless man. Neither is it a very far-fetched inference that a man who inherits one article of such value is pretty well provided for in other respects."

I nodded to show that I followed his reasoning.

"It is very customary for pawnbrokers in England, when they take a watch, to scratch the numbers of the ticket with a pin-point upon the inside of the case. It is more handy than a label as there is no risk of the number being lost or transposed. There are no less than four such numbers visible to my lens on the inside of this case. Inference—that your brother was often at low water. Secondary inference—that he had occasional bursts of prosperity, or he could not have redeemed the pledge. Finally, I ask you to look at the inner plate, which contains the keyhole. Look at the thousands of scratches all round the hole—marks where the key has slipped. What sober man's key could have scored those grooves? But you will never see a drunkard's watch without them. He winds it at night, and he leaves these traces of his unsteady hand. Where is the mystery in all this?"

"It is as clear as daylight," I answered. "I regret the injustice which I did you. I should have had more faith in your marvelous faculty."

This classic dialogue between fictional characters Sherlock Holmes and his sidekick Dr. Watson comes from chapter 1 of Sir Arthur Conan Doyle's *The Sign of the Four*, first published in 1890.

Legendary Detectives in Fiction (and Their Authors)

Porfiry Petrovich (Fyodor Dostoevsky)
Sherlock Holmes (Sir Arthur Conan Doyle)
Hercule Poirot (Agatha Christie)
Miss Jane Marple (Agatha Christie)
Charlie Chan (Earl Derr Biggers)
C. Auguste Dupin (Edgar Allan Poe)
Father Brown (Gilbert Keith [G. K.] Chesterton)
Nero Wolfe (Rex Stout)
Ellery Queen (Ellery Queen, pseudonym for Frederic Dannay and
 Manfred B. Lee)

This story, and others like it in *The Adventures of Sherlock Holmes* series, was written and published over a century ago, yet Holmes's ability to "profile" the watch owner in this excerpt used techniques similar to those profilers use today. He studied the evidence, and that evidence provided clues about the person who owned the watch. Though psychology wasn't part of Holmes's skill set, the fictional detective reached conclusions about the previous owner of the watch by using common sense, logic, and attention to detail.

In this case, the fictional character's profiling technique accurately reflects many of the techniques used by modern profilers: a combination of observation, knowledge, experience, logic, and reasoning. The advantage today's profilers have is their additional knowledge of psychology, a tool unavailable to Sherlock Holmes in the late nineteenth century. Still, Holmes's "profile" of Dr. Watson's brother well illustrates how real profilers use factual, hard evidence to make assumptions about people.

Just as Sir Arthur Conan Doyle used investigative techniques in his works that were popular in his time, today's novelists, playwrights, and scriptwriters have their characters use current investigative procedures and technologies.

Profiling in Modern Fiction

Many of today's popular novelists use profilers or profiling in their fiction: Thomas Harris created FBI trainee Clarice Starling in *The Silence of the Lambs* and FBI profiler Will Graham in *Red Dragon*; Edward X. Delaney used Detective Lawrence Sanders in *The Third Deadly Sin*; James Patterson calls on forensic psychologist Alex Cross in *Kiss the Girls*; Caleb Carr uses Dr. Laszlo Kriezler to get inside the head of the killer in *The Alienist* and *The Angel of Darkness*; and author John Sanford supplies the reader with Detective Lucas Davenport to develop profiles in *Chosen Prey*, *Secret Prey*, *Certain Prey*, and other works in his *Prey* series.

Novelists aren't the only fiction writers who use criminal psychology and profiling: television and movie writers have been using these techniques for decades. In addition to television shows like *Law & Order* (and its related shows), *CSI* (and its spin-offs), *Profiler* (in syndication), and *Medium* (a 2005 addition), movies like *Manhunter* (1986), *The Silence of the Lambs* (1991), *Basic Instinct* (1992), *Seven* (1995), *Hannibal* (2001), and

Red Dragon (2002), and *Mindhunters* (2004) have popularized profiling and its use in law enforcement.

While most authors and screenwriters attempt to accurately reflect contemporary standards and protocols for true investigative profiling (and they often get it right), virtually all of them and their classic-literature cousins from decades past fall short in one regard: in fiction, the profile always works, and the criminal is always exposed (though not always brought to justice). Real-life profiling doesn't work that way.

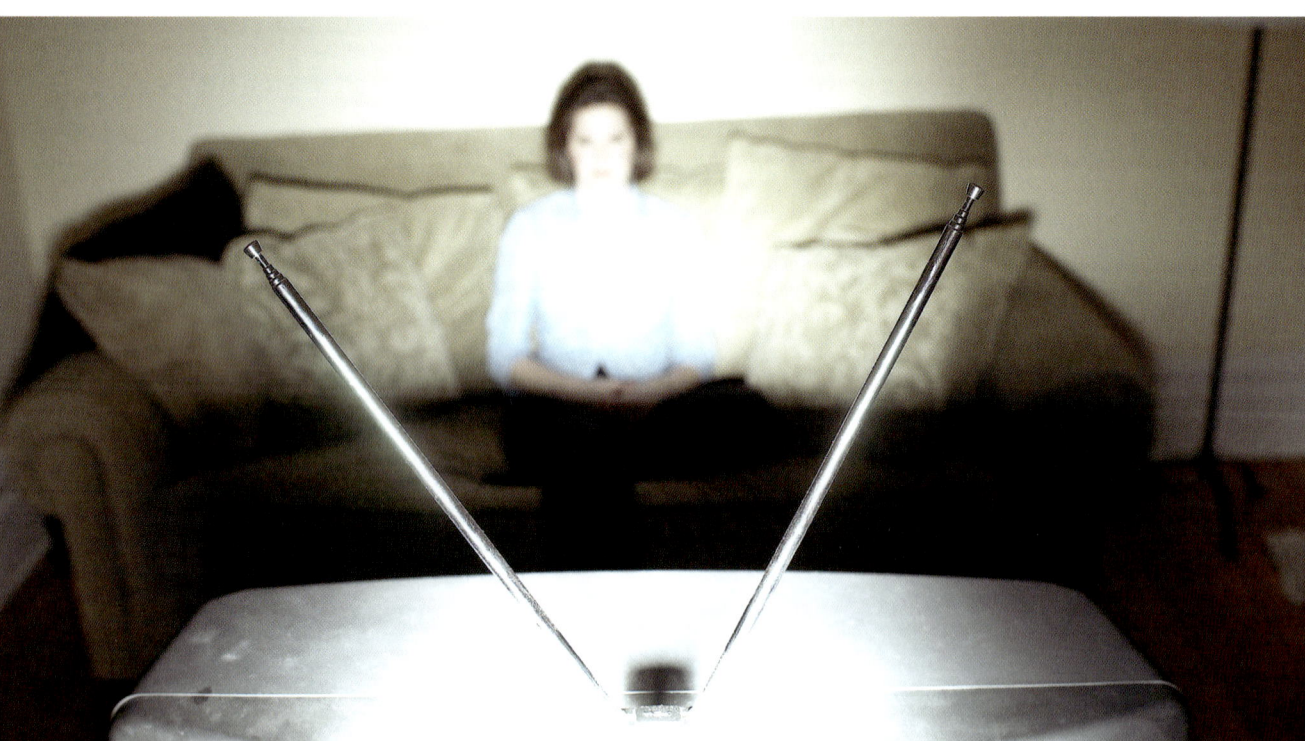

The use of criminal psychology to solve crimes is often seen on television. In real life, it's not as easy or as clear cut as it might seem on television and film.

Real-Life Profiling in History: Adolf Hitler

During the 1940s, North Americans were heavily engaged in World War II, and Adolf Hitler became archenemy number one—the most wanted criminal in the freedom-loving world. In 1942, the U.S. government formed an intelligence agency called the Office of Strategic Services (OSS) to coordinate with other federal agencies and to perform special operations related to winning the war. In 1943, the OSS hired a psychiatrist, Dr. Walter C. Langer, to develop an appraisal—essentially a profile—of Adolf Hilter: his ambitions, his reasons for invading neighboring countries, his power, his psychological makeup, his mental state, possible future behaviors, and possible means of his demise.

Langer's profile included predictions and observations: Hitler would make progressively fewer public appearances as his power diminished; he would grow increasingly paranoid, even suspecting his closest associates; he would grow more enraged; and his mental condition would further deteriorate. When Langer prepared his profile, he wanted to provide military officials with information that would either help them develop a workable way to interrogate someone they viewed as a madman if he were captured, or that would help them make future decisions regarding actions taken in war.

Unlike profiles in fiction, Langer's profile didn't lead to the desired outcomes of Hitler's capture, interrogation, or even to wartime decision making or strategizing based on the information contained within the profile. History, however, verifies that Langer's profile of Hitler's possible outcomes was startlingly correct. As he neared defeat, Adolf Hitler committed suicide in a bunker in Berlin in April 1945, and his final writings indicated that his mental condition was becoming increasingly fragile.

Excerpts from Dr. Walter C. Langer's Profile of Adolf Hitler

1. Hitler may die of natural cause.
2. Hitler might seek refuge in a neutral country.
3. Hitler might get killed in battle.
4. Hitler might be assassinated.
5. Hitler may go insane.
6. German military might revolt and seize him.
7. Hitler may fall into enemy hands.
8. Hitler might commit suicide (the most plausible outcome).

(Source: Ronald M. Holmes and Stephen T. Holmes, *Profiling Violent Crimes: An Investigative Tool*, 3rd edition)

A Historic Profiling Failure: The Boston Strangler

Langer's profile was correct, but it didn't lead to the successful capture or interrogation of the subject. In the case of the Boston Strangler, profilers appear to have gotten the profile wrong.

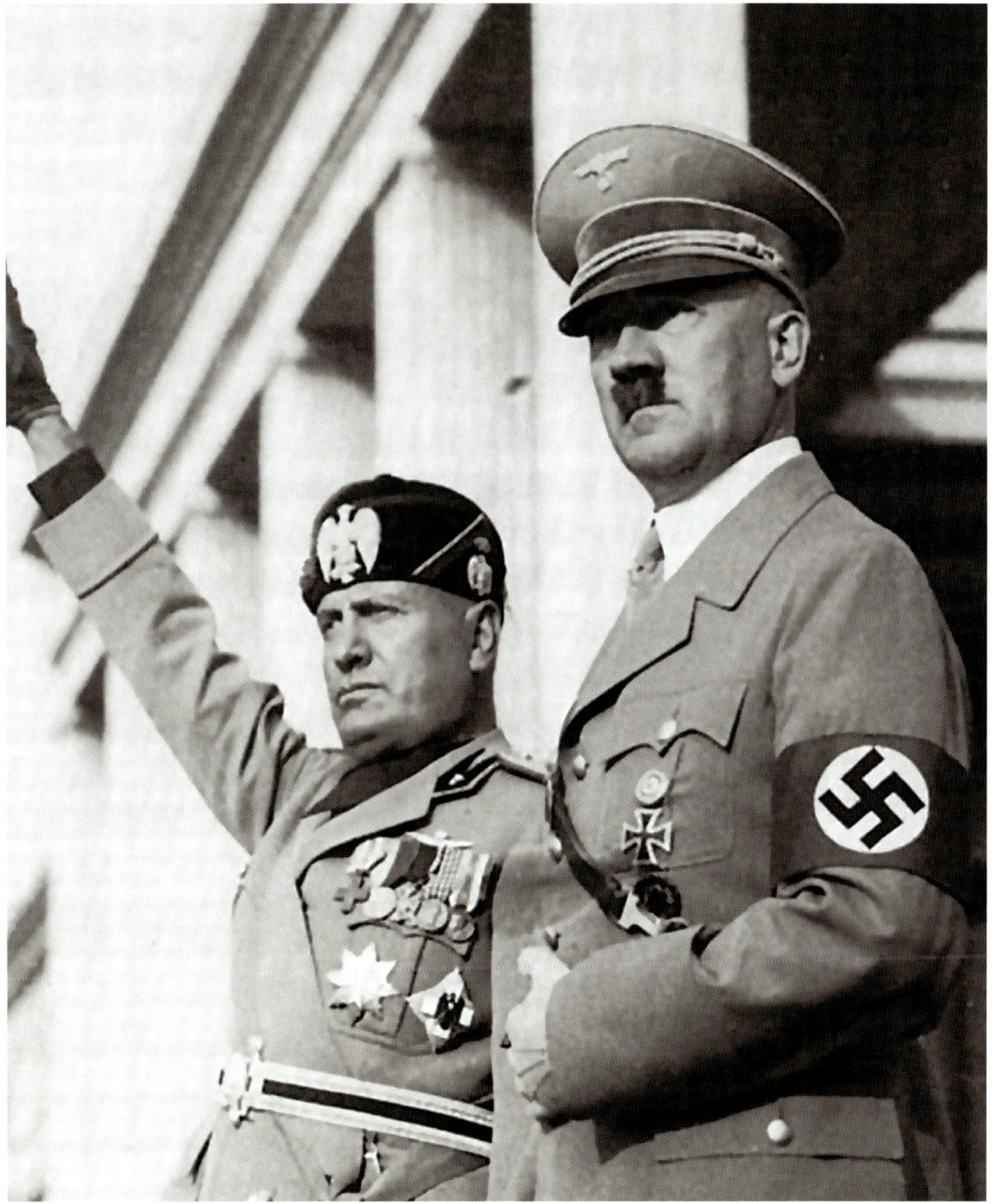

Adolf Hitler (right)

Criminal Profiling in Fiction and History

Case Study:
The Boston Strangler

Although Albert DeSalvo confessed to the Boston Strangler murders, the prosecution was unable to establish enough evidence that he had committed these crimes. No one was ever charged in the Boston Strangler killings, though many felt the true perpetrator was in prison.

More than thirty-five years after the last Boston Strangler murder, the final victim, Mary Sullivan, was exhumed from her grave. A semen stain on her body was tested for DNA. Although no nuclear DNA had survived the intervening years, scientists did find mitochondrial DNA. Investigators used blood from Albert DeSalvo's brother, Richard, to get a sample of mitochondrial DNA, which would be identical to Albert DeSalvo's since it is passed through the maternal line. Instead of confirming that DeSalvo was Sullivan's killer, as many expected, the tests revealed that the semen did not belong to DeSalvo, making it far less likely he had committed the crime.

Between June of 1962 and January of 1964, women in Boston, Massachusetts, fell prey to a serial murderer who sexually assaulted and strangled his victims. In all, the serial killer murdered thirteen women. All lived in the Boston metro area; most were older women; all were strangled, usually with a piece of their own clothing; all had been sadistically sexually assaulted;

and in each case, the killer provided his unique "signature"—a neat bow tied beneath the victim's chin.

With growing panic among Boston's citizens, state authorities appointed a panel to develop a profile of the suspect. These experts included, among others, a psychiatrist with knowledge of sex crimes, a physician with experience in anthropology, a gynecologist, and Dr. James Brussels, the famous psychiatrist who'd so accurately developed the profile of New York City's Mad Bomber in 1956.

The panel was divided. Most panel members felt the thirteen murders under review were committed not by one but two perpetrators. Both perpetrators were thought to be unmarried, had weak or distant fathers, were sexually inadequate, and hated their deceased but once-abusive mothers. One perpetrator lived alone and killed the older women; the other might have been a homosexual who knew and killed the younger women.

Brussels disagreed. He believed all thirteen murders were committed by the same person who changed his MO. He felt the perpetrator didn't fit either profile provided by the rest of the committee. Rather, he thought the serial killer was probably of Spanish or Italian heritage, would be at least thirty years old, and that over the two-year killing spree the murderer had "grown psychosexually from infancy to puberty to manhood." Evidence for this "growth" came from the fact that the Strangler left his fourteenth victim alive; he assaulted her and then apologized for his crime.

That victim was able to provide a description of her attacker to the police, which led to the arrest of thirty-three-year-old Albert DeSalvo. DeSalvo didn't even remotely fit the profiles provided by the special profiling committee: He was married; his wife said he had a voracious sexual appetite; he fathered two children; he had criminal records for child molestation, breaking and entering, and burglary. After his arrest, he claimed to have raped more than 300 women in the New England area as

Criminal Profiling in Fiction and History **77**

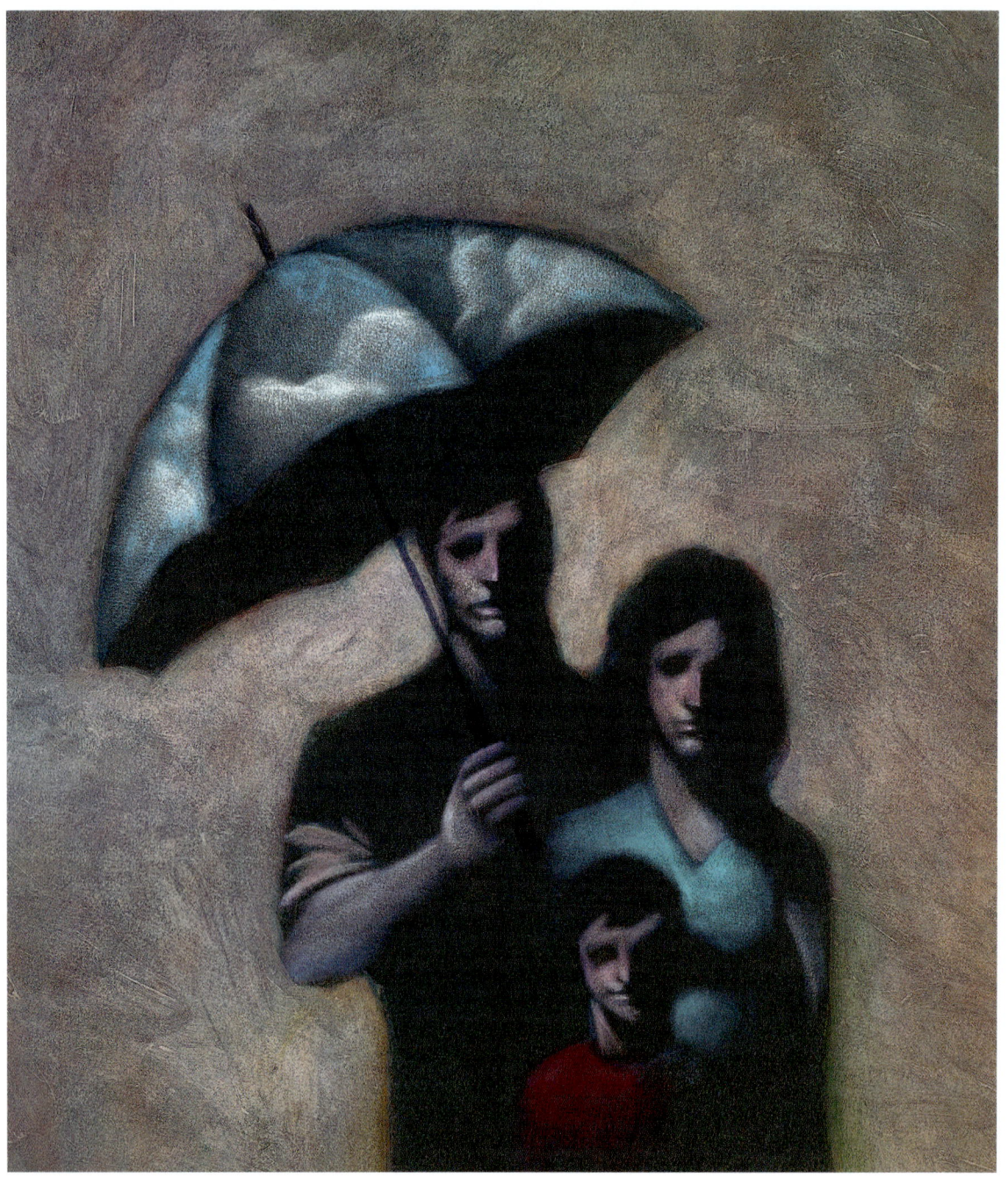

The Boston Strangler was not the loner investigators profiled him to be; he had a wife and family.

an offender known as the "Green Man." He also confessed to the Boston Strangler murders, as well as two more. Police and mental health professionals found his confessions to be credible because he provided details that had never been made public—ones only the killer could know.

In 1965, after being diagnosed as a schizophrenic, DeSalvo was detained indefinitely for observation. Then, in 1967, a jury convicted him of the "Green Man" break-ins and sentenced him to life in prison. DeSalvo was murdered by another inmate in 1973.

Unlike what is portrayed in the movies, the Boston Strangler profile failed to lead to an arrest and conviction. This failure gave profiling a bad name for the next several years. It wasn't until the successful use of profiling in another famous case in the early 1970s that profiling became a credible tool in law enforcement once again.

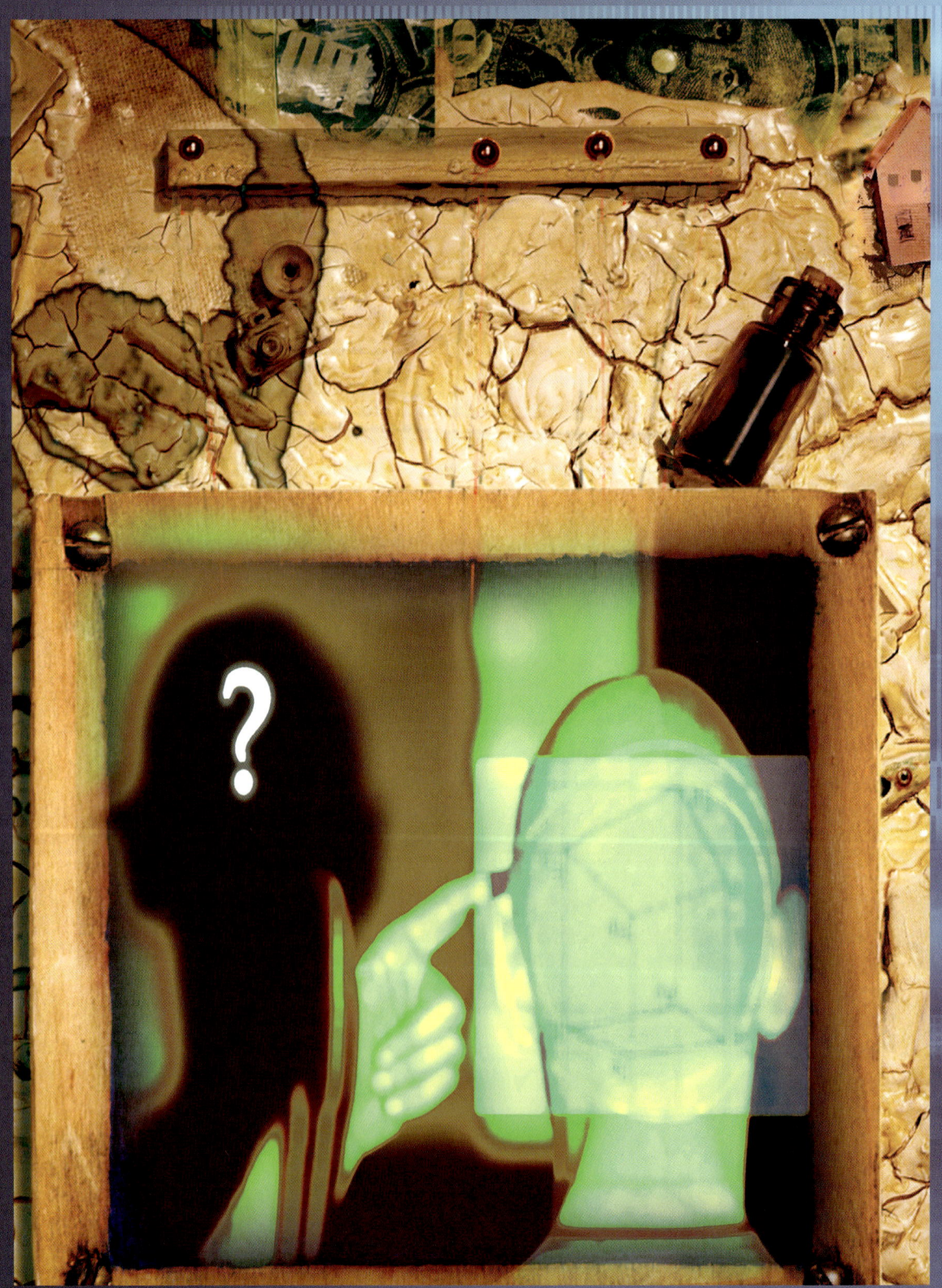

5

CRIME-SPECIFIC PROFILING

Over half (57%) of . . . child abduction murders are committed by a killer who is a stranger to the victim. Family involvement in this type of case is infrequent (9%). However, the relationship between the victim and the killer varies with the gender and age of the victim. The youngest females, 1–5 years old, tend to be killed by friends or acquaintances (64%), while the oldest females, 16–17 years old, tend to be killed by strangers (also 64%). The relationship between the killer and victim is different for the male victims. The youngest male victims (1–5 years old) are most likely to be killed by strangers (also 64%), as are the teenage males (13–15 years old, 60% and 16–17 years old, 58%).

The average age of killers of abducted children is around 27 years old. They are predominantly unmarried (85%) and half of them (51%) either live alone (17%)

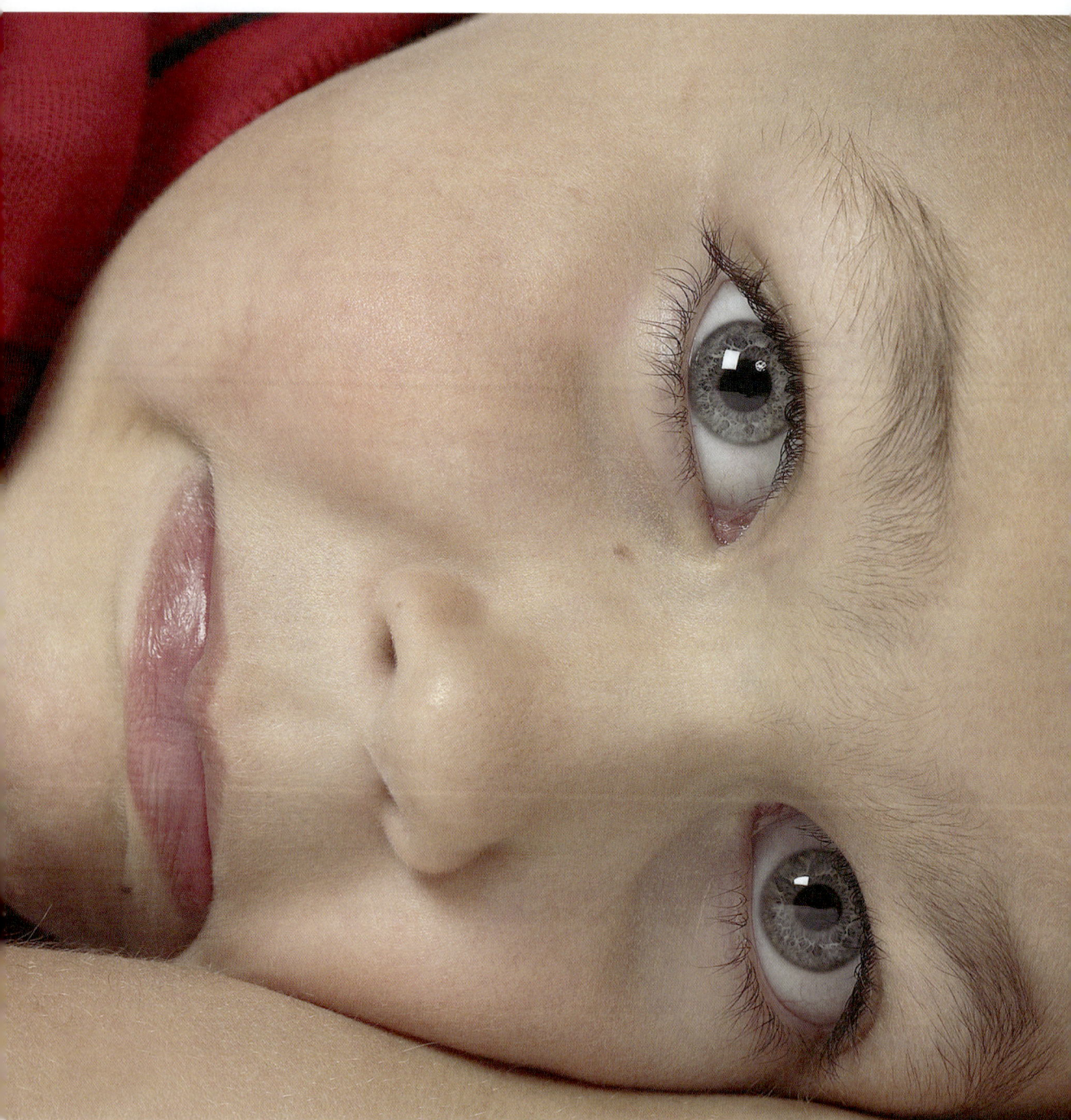

Criminals who prey on young people take advantage of children's innocence and vulnerability.

CRIMINAL PSYCHOLOGY & PERSONALITY PROFILING

or with their parents (34%). Half of them are unemployed, and those that are employed work in unskilled or semi-skilled labor occupations. Therefore, the killers can generally be characterized as "social marginals."

Almost two-thirds of the killers (61%) had prior arrests for violent crimes, with slightly more than half of the killers' prior crimes (53%) committed against children. The most frequent prior crimes against children were rape (31% of killers) and other sexual assault (45% of killers). Sixty-seven percent of the child abduction murderers' prior crimes were similar in M.O. to the murder that was committed by the same killer.

Commonly, the killers are at the initial victim-killer contact site for a legitimate reason (66%). They either lived in the area (29%) or were engaging in some normal activity. Most of the victims of child abduction murder are victims of opportunity (57%). Only in 14 percent of cases did the killer choose his victim because of some physical characteristic of the victim. The primary motivation for the child abduction murder is sexual assault.

The above profile of child-abductor-homicide perpetrators and victims is quoted from a report titled *Case Management for Missing Children Homicide Investigation*, created jointly by Washington's attorney general Christine O. Gregoire and the U.S. Department of Justice's Office of Juvenile Justice and Delinquency Prevention. This public document illustrates how criminal profiling can help law enforcement officials find criminals and equip the public to protect themselves.

By using profiles specific to the crime of child-abduction murder, law enforcement officials dealing with a missing or murdered child have a place from which they can begin to develop theories about the perpetrator. Other profiles—for example, those of serial murderers, rapists, or arsonists—won't match the profile of a child-abductor murderer. Investigators need information about offenders specific to certain crimes.

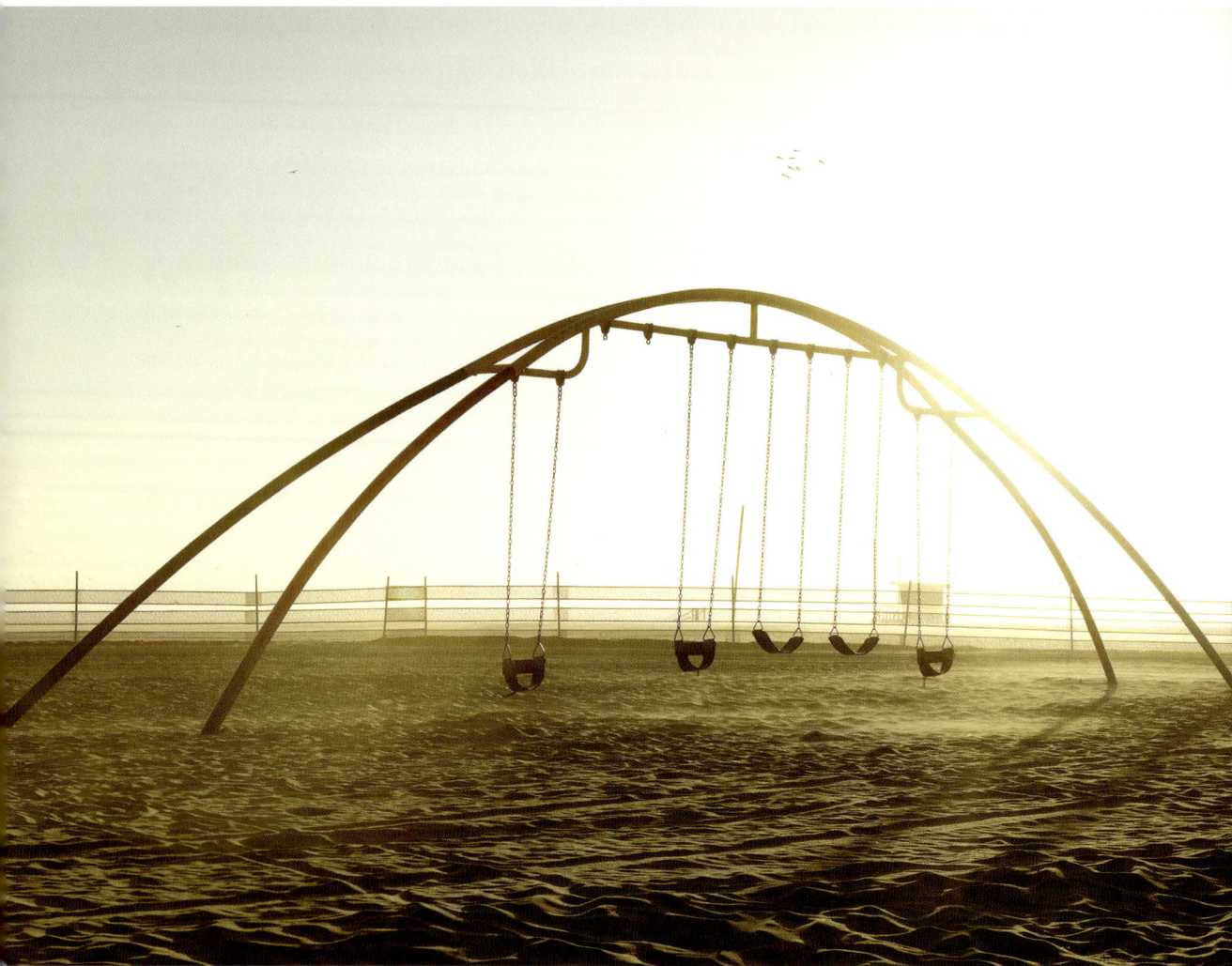

During the Atlanta Child Murders, parents would not leave their children unattended.

After the failure of profiling in the Boston-Strangler case in the early 1960s, law enforcement stayed away from using profiles for many years. It wasn't until the early 1970s that criminal psychologists and law enforcement officials began developing profiles once again. The case that brought crime-specific profiling back in vogue was the Atlanta child-serial-murder investigation.

The Atlanta Child Murders: Profiling Returns

When police detectives received a call about a foul odor in a wooded area off of Niskey Lake Road outside Atlanta, Georgia, in 1979, they had no idea

When Is a Murderer Considered a Serial Killer?

According to the FBI's Crime Classification Manual, for someone to be considered a "serial killer," he or she must have committed "three or more separate events (murders) in three or more separate locations with an emotional cooling-off period in between." By emphasizing the number of murders, their locations, and their differences in timing, the FBI distinguishes serial killing from other types of crime. For example, an angry student kills multiple people at school by setting off a bomb in his locker during the time when classes change. While his crime meets the minimum-number-of-victims requirement (three or more) for serial killings, it doesn't meet the place and time requirements provided in the FBI's definition. The student's killings happened at the same time in the same place. This crime would be called mass murder.

Fast Fact:

Hit men, hired assassins, terrorists, and politically motivated murderers are not classified as serial killers.

the result of that call would throw the city and its citizens into a full-blown, two-year nightmare. Police investigated the site and found two decomposing bodies: one of thirteen-year-old Alfred Evans and the other of fourteen-year-old Edward Smith. Both had been missing for a week or less. These two teenagers were the first of what would become twenty-nine murders over the next two years. All the victims were black; all but two were male; and they ranged in age from eight to twenty-seven years, though most were in their early teens. The media labeled the serial killings the Atlanta Child Murders, and the killings kept Atlanta's citizens in a state of high alert bordering on panic.

Parents feared for their children's safety as they walked to school or went out to play; many parents refused to let their children be outside without an adult. Law enforcement officials were frustrated as someone killed Atlanta's children—seemingly without fear of being caught. Investigators knew they had a serial killer in their city, but they didn't know who it was. They needed help. An incident halfway through the string of murders proved to be the break law enforcement needed.

After ten-year-old Earl Terrell disappeared in July 1980, his parents received several telephone calls demanding ransom from an *alleged* kidnapper who claimed to have taken their son from Georgia to Alabama. The fact

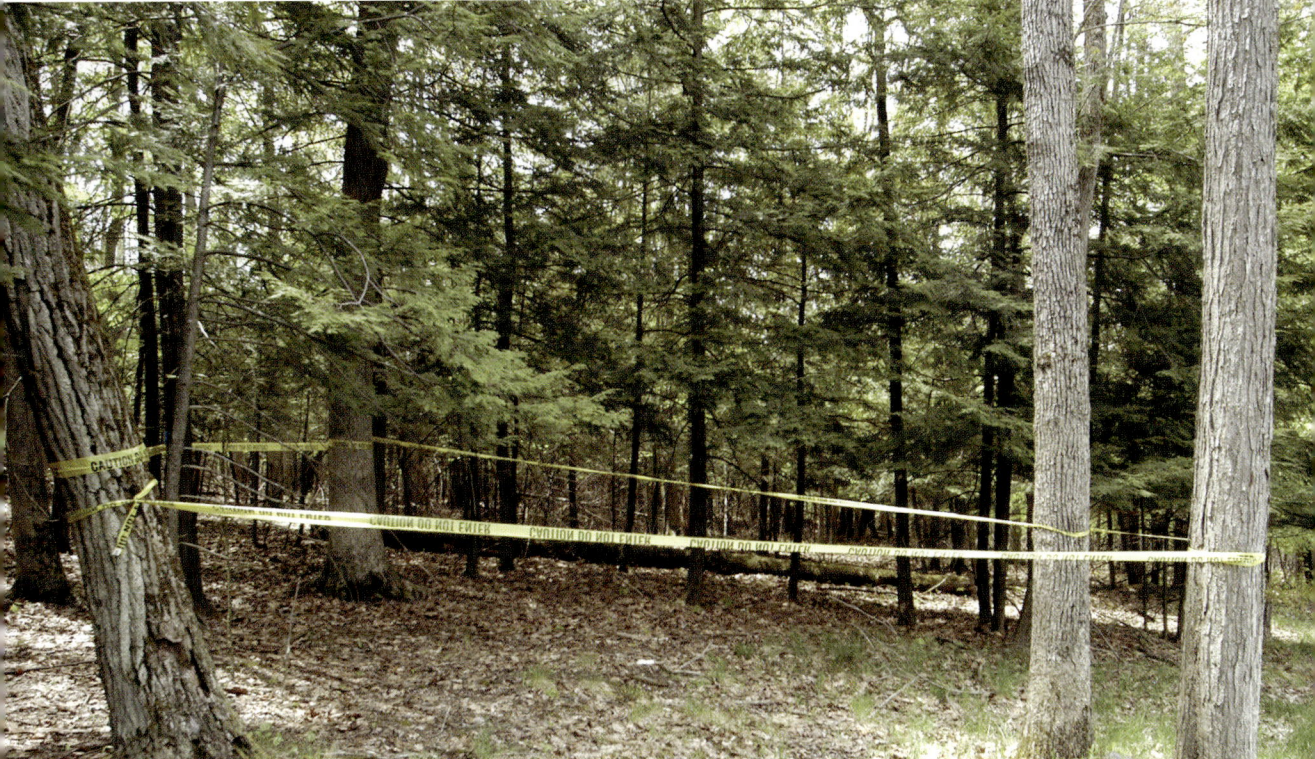

The Atlanta Child Murderer's first victims were discovered in the woods.

that the victim was supposedly taken across state lines moved the case (and all cases related to it) from local and state jurisdiction to federal jurisdiction. That meant the FBI could become involved. When the telephone calls proved to be a hoax, then–Attorney General Griffin Bell ordered the FBI to look into the cases of the missing children. Was it possible that they had been taken across state lines?

FBI agents and BSU instructors Roy Hazelwood and John Douglas were sent to Atlanta. The two reviewed the case files: crime-scene photos, details about how the victims were dressed, how the autopsies had been conducted, and statements from police interviews. The two seasoned de-

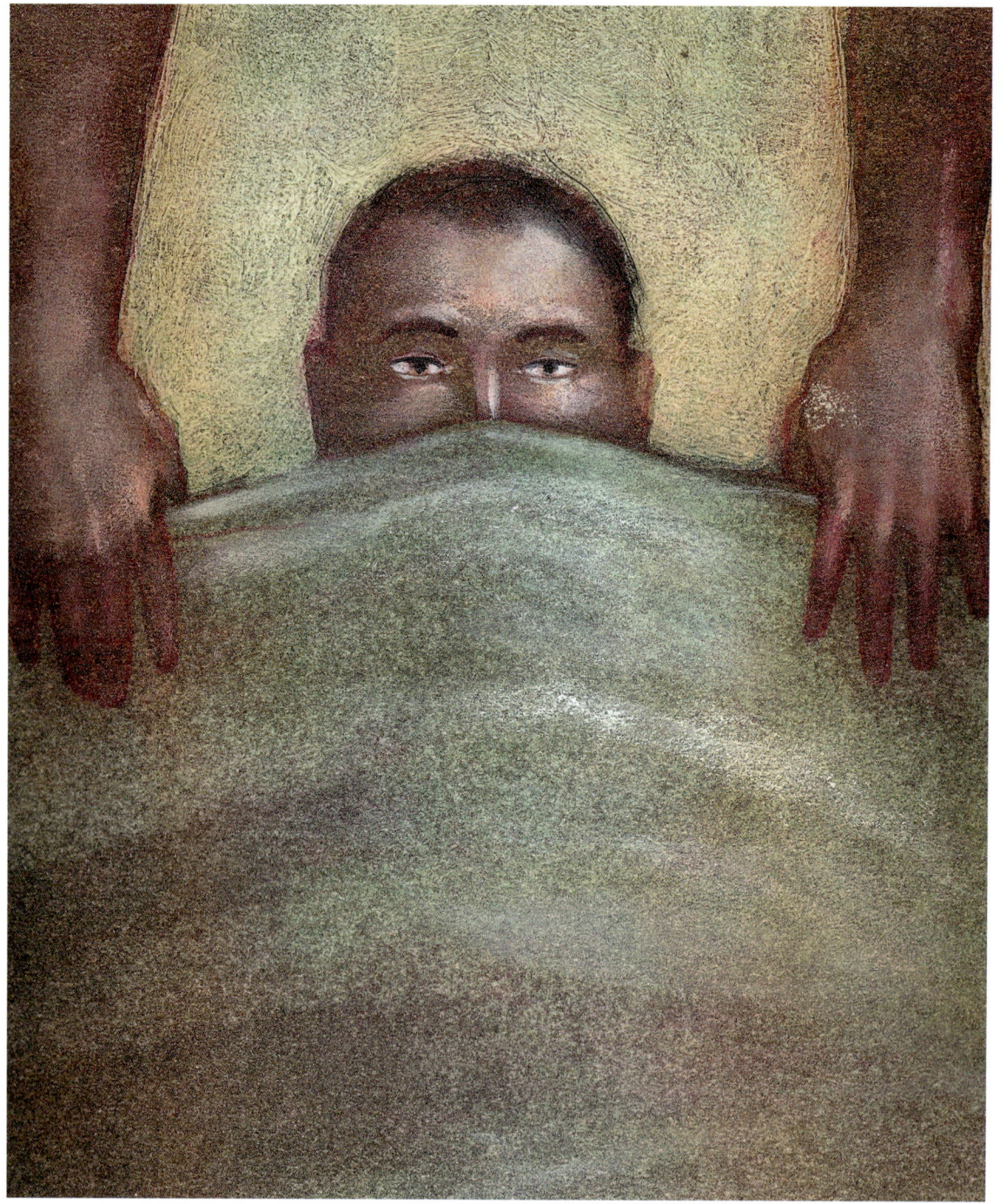

Investigators created a profile to "uncover" specific traits of the killer.

Not an Exact Science

The work of the profilers in the Boston Strangler case was completely wrong. The profile compiled in the Atlanta Child Murders was completely right. Or were they?

DNA evidence in the Boston Strangler case casts doubt on the guilt of Albert DeSalvo. In 2005, the cases of five of the murdered Atlanta children were reopened. Wayne Williams was not convicted of murdering any of those children, and the DeKalb County Chief of Police believes that Williams murdered no one. So, although he might have fit the profile, it is possible Williams is innocent.

Does this mean that profiles aren't useful? Of course not. But they should be considered as just one part of an investigation.

tectives examined the victims' backgrounds and interviewed their family members to see what the victims had in common. They visited where the bodies had been dumped. They examined the neighborhoods where each of the children disappeared. After careful analysis, they summarized their findings into what they believed was an accurate profile of the killer. What they came up with differed from what many people expected. John Douglas describes their profile in detail in his book *Mindhunter: Inside the FBI's Elite Serial Crime Unit*. What follows is adapted from that account.

First, because all the victims were black and came from predominantly black areas of the city, the two profilers felt the perpetrator must be black. How else could he move easily in and out of the victims' neighborhoods

Crimes Best Suited to Profiling

Not every crime is the kind in which a profile of an unknown subject is beneficial. Vernon J. Geberth, retired lieutenant-commander of the New York City Police Department and author of the "homicide-investigation bible" Practical Homicide Investigation: Tactics, Procedures, and Forensic Techniques, suggests that these crimes are most suitable for profiling:

- serial rapes
- sexual assaults that include sadistic torture
- murders related to sex or lust
- murders in which internal organs have been removed or revealed
- murders in which the bodies were mutilated after death
- crimes involving the occult
- pedophilia and other forms of sexual abuse of children
- terroristic letter writings and threats
- obscene letter writings and threats
- arsons that appear to have no motive

without drawing attention to himself? Both agents knew from experience that most sexual killers (the Atlanta Child Murders fit a sexual-murder pattern) target their own race.

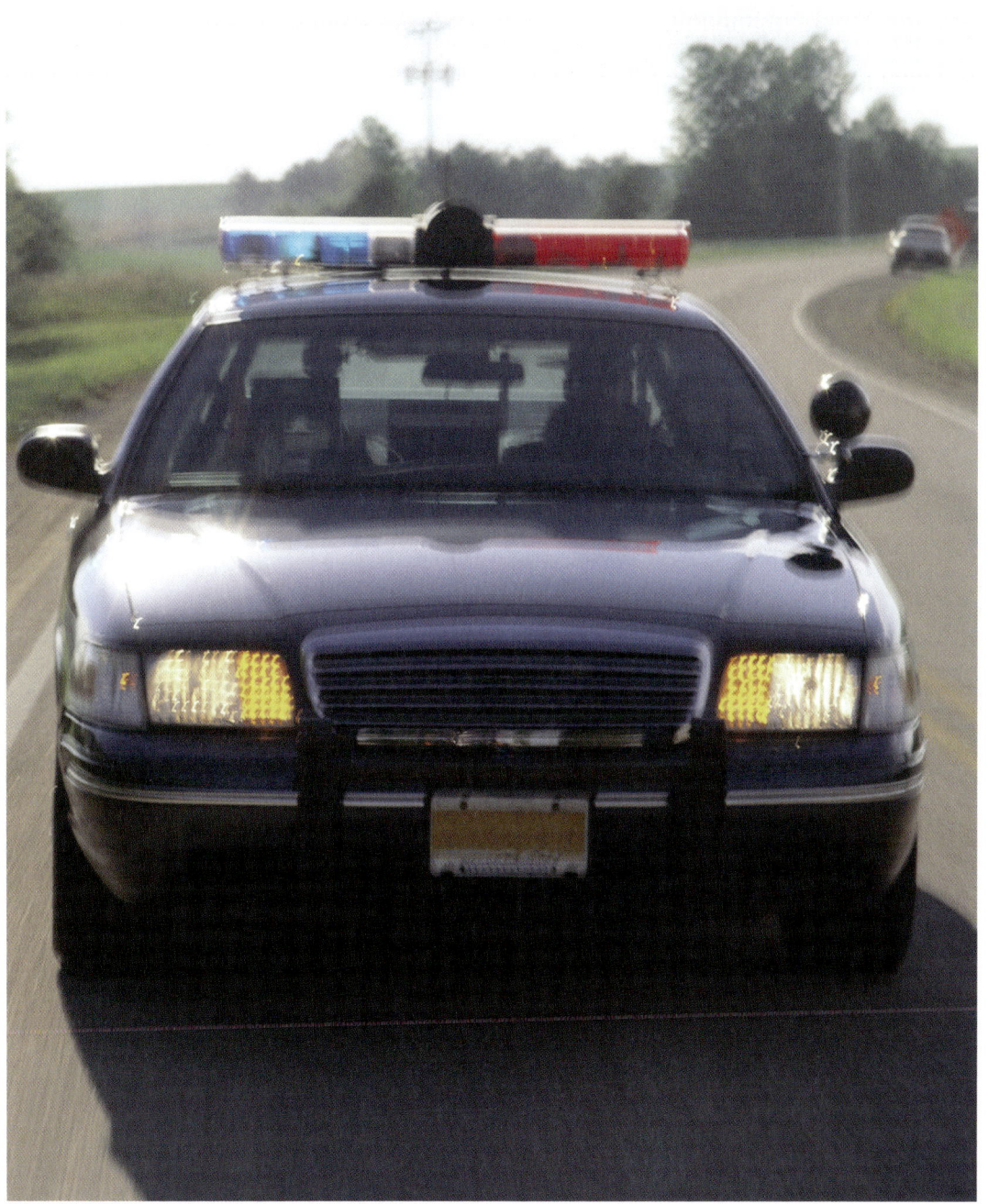

The Atlanta Child murderer had to gain the trust of his victims. He used a police-type car to lure children.

One Way to Categorize Serial Killers

Dr. Kim Rossmo, a detective inspector in Vancouver, British Columbia, developed a way to categorize serial killers based on how they find their victims:

the Hunter
the Poacher
the Troller
the Trapper
the Raptor
the Stalker
the Ambusher

Second, Hazelwood and Douglas felt the perpetrator had to have a car; the children had all been taken from where they were abducted and transported elsewhere. The profilers also believed the car would be a police-type vehicle, perhaps even a car that had once been used by law enforcement.

They offered several other details about their idea of who was committing these crimes: He would be single and in his mid- to late twenties. He would be a police buff and might have impersonated an officer. He would own a police-type dog. He would not have a girlfriend. He would have some kind of talent or trick he would use to lure his victims into talking with him—probably something to do with music. He would be following the case's development in the press and would react to developments he saw

Fast Fact:

Most experts agree that the number of serial murders and of serial murderers in North America is unknown. Estimates range from a low of twenty to as high as three hundred.

there. As evidence mounted, he would start dumping bodies in the river to destroy any possible future evidence that could be used against him.

The details of this profile prompted police officers to begin watching for suspicious activity around bridges and rivers. One officer on surveillance saw a car drive across the Jackson Parkway Bridge, which spanned the Chattahoochee River, stop briefly in the middle, turn around, and come back across the bridge. After the car stopped but before it turned around, the officer heard a big splash.

The surveillance officer pulled over the suspicious car. The driver was a light-skinned black man named Wayne Bertram Williams. Without sufficient cause to arrest him, the police let him go, but they kept their eyes on him. As it turned out, Wayne Williams matched the FBI profile almost completely: he was black; he owned a car; he owned a German Shepherd; he was a police buff; he'd been arrested for impersonating an officer; he was twenty-three years old; he was single; and he presented himself as a "music-biz talent scout."

When a body was found floating in the Chattahoochee River two days after the surveillance officer stopped Williams, police arrested Wayne Williams and charged him with murder. Investigators found hair and fiber evidence in Williams's car that directly linked him to twelve of the Atlanta murders. Eyewitnesses put him with one of the victims. His German Shepherd's hair was found on the body of one of the victims. In January 1982, he was tried and found guilty of the last two murders and sentenced to life in prison. The murders stopped after his arrest.

Though solid investigation and fiber analysis are what provided the hard evidence prosecutors needed to convict the Atlanta Child Murderer, law enforcement officials credit the profile provided by FBI agents Hazelwood and Douglas as the critical tool that turned the investigation around. The accuracy of their profile also did much to help law enforcement officials and the judiciary to once again embrace profiling as a legitimate tool in the arsenal of criminal investigation and prosecution.

Profiling Since Atlanta

Since the FBI's success in Atlanta in the early 1980s, profiling has come a long way. Experts in the field have developed generalized profiles for perpetrators of different kinds. Serial arsonists, researchers have discovered, generally fit one profile. Serial rapists fit another. Sexual sadists fit a third. Occult-related crime sprees require a different profile from the rest. How profiles are developed and the kind of profile used depends on the type of crime itself, and then on the specifics of that crime.

Serial killers have their own classifications and characteristics. One classification developed by Hazelwood and Douglas divides all serial killers into two groups based on how they commit their crimes: organized or disorganized. (For more on organized and disorganized offenders, refer back to chapter 3.) Another way to profile serial killers is based on how they choose their victims. Did the murderer pick her ahead of time and stalk her the way a cheetah would stalk a gazelle? Did the offender pick his victim spontaneously by random selection? Or did the victim just happen to be in the wrong place at the wrong time?

Today, most law enforcement officials have access to standardized profiles of offenders for various crimes. While these profiles suggest what an offender *might* be like or how an offender will *most likely* behave, they are incomplete pictures at best. Profiling, no matter how far it has come, is still only one resource available to investigators among a host of forensic investigative techniques.

Profiling alone doesn't solve crimes; it's only when pro-filing is used in conjunction with other sound investigative procedures that cases are successfully solved. But because profiling has been so successful in a few high-profile cases, some investigators rely too much on profiling and not enough on old-fashioned detective work and sound evidence-gathering techniques. This is only one danger inherent in the use of criminal psychology and profiling to combat crime. There are more.

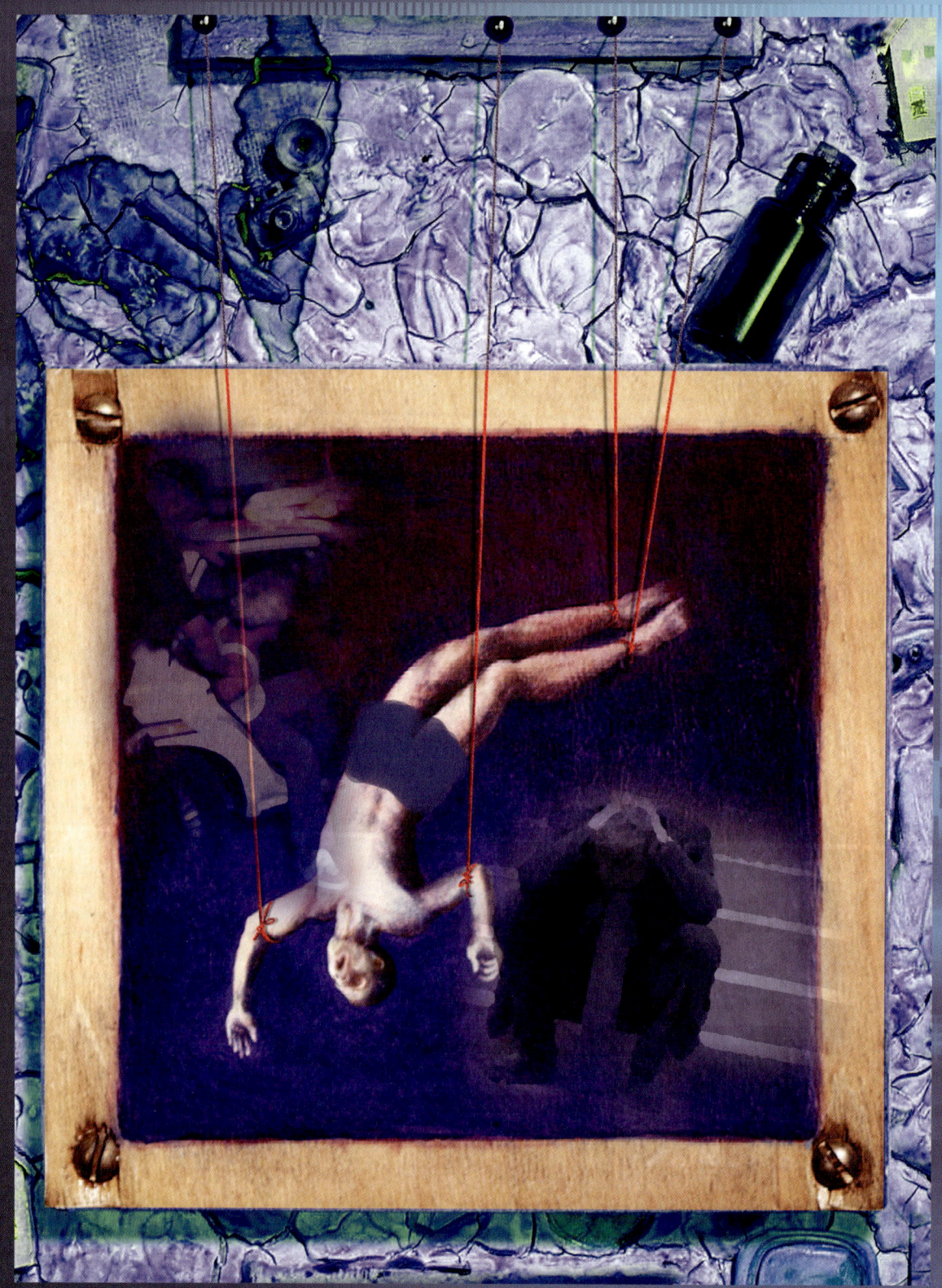

6

THE DANGERS, TEMPTATIONS, AND LIMITATIONS OF CRIMINAL PSYCHOLOGY

Criminal psychologists and profilers face many dangers in their professions.

- One agent is killed on the job.
- Another develops stress-related illnesses.
- One is assaulted by a subject during an interview.
- A fourth alienates his peers by focusing too narrowly on his profile.
- Another agent can no longer sympathize with his children's normal, everyday hurts because of the extreme suffering he's seen some children experience at the hands of criminals.

- An agent loses his marriage when his wife can no longer handle the stress of her husband's job.
- Still others are seduced by their success and become overconfident, damaging their skills and reputations.
- Countless more burn out and find other jobs.
- Some make mistakes, and people die as a result.

These issues are just "part of the job" for criminal psychologists and profilers. Codes of ethics, interview protocols, peer support, vacations, friendships, religious faith, counseling, delegation of work, security measures, training, and education can help those in these fields navigate these hazards, but in the war on crime, some soldiers—especially those in law enforcement—experience various types of casualties or become casualties themselves.

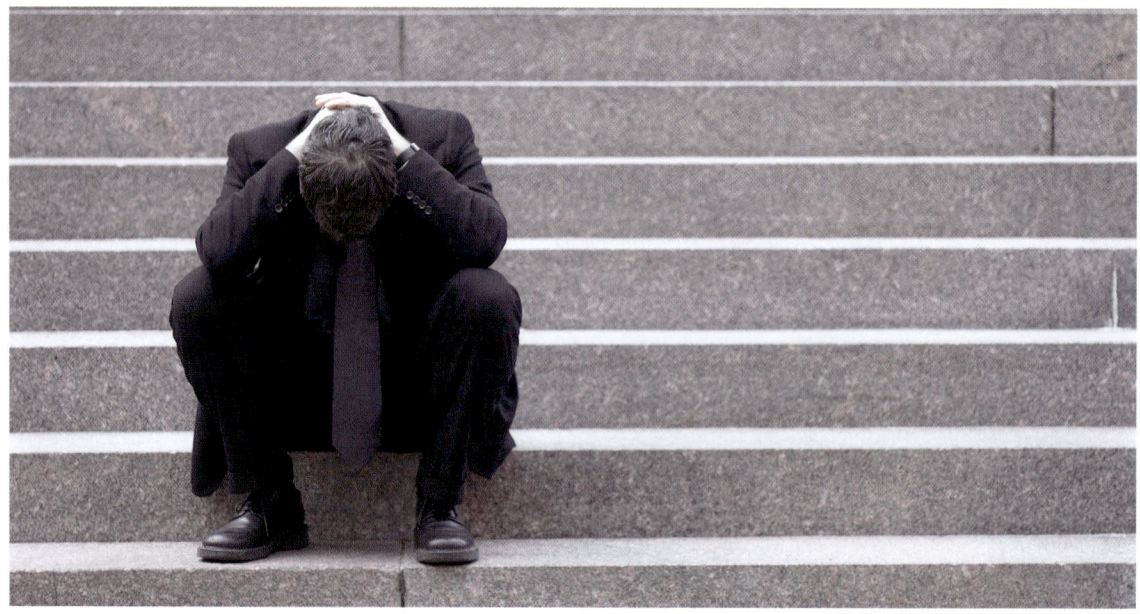

Criminal psychologists experience many emotional stressors.

For the criminal psychologist and profiler, the costs are often emotional or psychological. Though these jobs are glamorized in the media, the tedious hours of research and long hours of examining horrendous crimes, combined with the stress of knowing your input could save or cost lives, makes the reality of these vocations far different from the solve-it-every-time-in-sixty-minutes ideal of television shows.

No matter how far criminal psychology and profiling move into the law enforcement realm, they will never provide the clear-cut, black-and-white answers found in evidence analysis. The fields continue to be subjective sciences.

Still Inexact

In his book *Journey into Darkness*, profiler John Douglas reminds readers:

> Life and death decisions can be made based on [our] advice, yet [we] don't have the luxury of hard facts to back them up . . . [our] stock-in-trade is human behavior, and human behavior, the psychiatrists are so fond of telling [us], is not an exact science.

Though criminal profiling has come a long way toward being accepted as a legitimate resource for investigators to use, it is still met with suspicion by some police departments and law enforcement agencies. This skepticism occurs in part because profiling is still an inexact science based on observations, instincts, and general patterns of behavior rather than on definitive evidence, formulas, and facts. Law enforcement officials sometimes still second-guess criminal psychologists.

In one investigation in 1993, New York City detectives, working on the case of a missing ten-year-old girl who was held captive in Long Island by a pedophile for seventeen days, blamed profiling for actually preventing them from solving the crime more quickly. Though the girl was eventually rescued, police complained that the profile provided for this case "distracted" and misled them because it stated that pedophiles don't hide their victims in their homes.

Some police officers still question the value of profiles. Others question whether criminal psychologists and profilers can be effective when many of the assessment tools psychologists use to evaluate criminals have limitations, and when only a handful of psychologists know how and when to best use them. If the people giving the tests are flawed, and the tests themselves are flawed, how can the results be anything but flawed?

Part of the problem is an expectation that profiling and criminal psychology solve crimes. But those in the field will tell you that they don't; they only add one piece to the crime-solving picture.

The mixed reception criminal psychologists and profilers receive in both the law enforcement world and the judicial system might be enough to dissuade someone from pursuing a career in either vocation. But for those who choose to assist crime solvers with psychology, the reward that comes with helping to solve a crime is well worth the criticism they may take from some peers. Sometimes, however, that reward is long in coming. In other cases, it never comes.

Not Every Crime Is Solved

- London's Jack the Ripper (1888)
- Lizzie Borden (1892)
- San Francisco's Zodiac killer (1966–1981)
- Canada's "Highway of Tears" Highway 16 in British Columbia (1990–2002)

- Edmonton, Alberta's prostitute slayings (1993–2004)
- Colorado's JonBenet Ramsey murder (1996)

These are just a few of the high-profile crimes that remain unsolved despite law enforcement's best attempts to find the perpetrators. At their best, they are intriguing case studies in human behavior; at their worst, they are glaring reminders of the limitations of criminal-investigation techniques, even today. Twenty-first century technology and evidence-processing techniques still aren't sufficient to solve every crime or identify every perpetrator. And when a person moves into law enforcement or the fields of criminal psy-

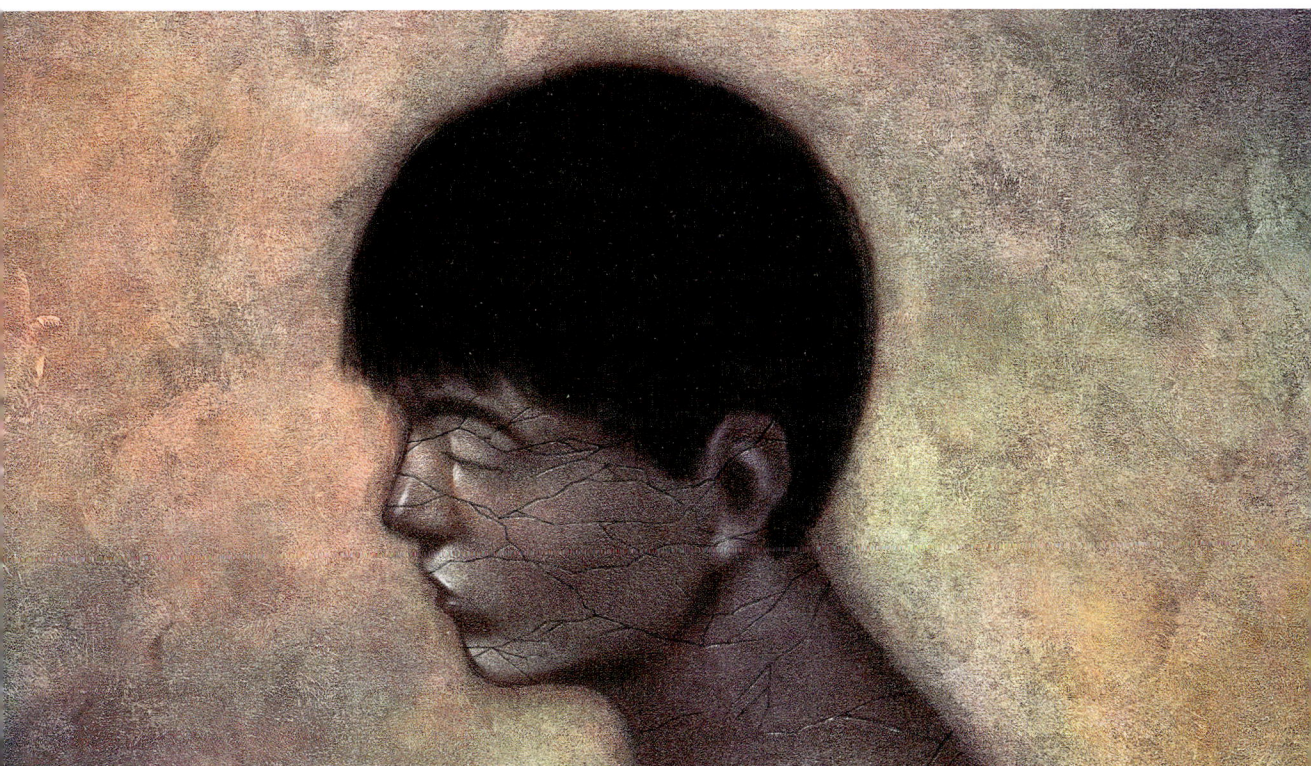

The horrors experienced in the field of criminal psychology are enough to force some agents to quit.

The Dangers and Limitations of Criminal Psychology

chology and profiling, he will have to adjust to the fact that not every crime can be solved.

For some investigators, that truth is tolerable. They can accept their limitations and move on, though a case may haunt them for years or decades. For others, the stress is too much to bear.

The Toll of Criminal Psychology and Profiling

In his book *Journey into Darkness*, twenty-five-year veteran of the FBI John Douglas describes what happened to him when the stress of dealing with horrific crime day-in and day-out finally caught up with him:

In early December of 1983, at thirty-eight years of age, I collapsed in a hotel room in Seattle while working on the Green River murders case. The two agents I'd brought with me from Quantico had to break down the door to get to me. For five days I hovered in a coma between life and death in the intensive care unit of Swedish Hospital suffering from viral encephalitis brought on by the acute stress of handling more than 150 cases at a time, all of which I knew were depending on me for answers.

I wasn't expected to live, but miraculously I did, nurtured by first-rate medical care, the love of my family, and the support of my fellow agents. I returned home, almost a month later, in a wheelchair and couldn't go back to work until May. All during that time I was afraid the neurological damage the disease left me with would prevent me from shooting at FBI standards and therefore permanently end my career as an agent. To this day, I still have some impairment on my left side.

Unfortunately, my situation isn't unique in this business. Most of the other agents who've worked with me as profilers and criminal investigative analysts . . . have suffered some severe, work-related stress or illness which kept them off the job for some period of time. The range of problems runs the gamut—neurological disease like mine, chest pain and cardiac scares, ulcers and GI (gastro-intestinal) disorders, anxieties and depression.

One of the greatest dangers faced by those who pursue careers in criminal psychology and profiling is the way it can adversely affect their personal lives and health. Retired chief of the FBI BSU Roger L. Depue, in his book Between Good and Evil, describes the cost paid by those who fight crime this way:

The task of fighting evil can take a terrible toll on the people who are charged with it. It can cost them their families, their equilibrium, their capacity for joy.

A relentless diet of human misery and sadistic violence can bring any human—even those armored by years of experience in a law enforcement career—to the brink of despair. I once came to that place myself. But I returned from it, because, along with the evil, I have also come to know something about the redemptive power of good.

That confidence, the confidence in the redemptive power of good as Depue calls it, is what draws people and allows them to persevere in the fields of criminal psychology and profiling.

Glossary

alleged: Claimed, but not yet proven.

atypical: Unusual, not typical.

auditory: Relating to hearing.

cavalierly: In a manner displaying arrogance or disregard, or with a carefree attitude.

charlatanism: The practice of falsely claiming a special skill or expertise.

credibility: The ability to inspire trust.

criminology: The sociological study of crime, criminals, and the punishment of criminals.

facets: Parts or aspects of something.

inferences: Conclusions drawn from evidence or reasoning.

linguistic: Relating to language or languages.

plausibility: Believability in the absence of proof.

pragmatic: Practical, concerned with facts.

precocious: More developed than is expected.

protocols: Standard procedures.

psychopathic: Possessing antisocial, aggressive, or perverted tendencies.

psychopathological: Relating to the study of the causes and development of psychiatric disorders.

sadists: People who achieve sexual satisfaction by causing pain in others.

schizophrenic: Having a psychotic disorder characterized by illogical thinking, hallucinations, delusions, and withdrawal from reality.

tangible: Real, capable of being touched or understood.

vogue: The state of being popular at a particular time.

voracious: Ravenous, insatiable.

Further Reading

Depue, Roger L., with Susan Schindehette. *Between Good and Evil: A Master Profiler's Hunt for Society's Most Violent Predators*. New York: Warner Books, 2005.

Douglas, John, and Mark Olshaker. *Mind Hunter: Inside the FBI's Elite Serial Crime Unit*. New York: Simon and Schuster, 1995.

Evans, Colin. *The Casebook of Forensic Detection: How Science Solved 100 of the World's Most Baffling Crimes*. New York: Berkley Books, 2007.

Holmes, Ronald M., and Stephen T. Holmes. *Profiling Violent Crimes: An Investigative Tool, Fourth Edition*. Thousand Oaks, Calif.: Sage Publications, 2008.

Innes, Brian. *Profile of a Criminal Mind: How Psychological Profiling Helps Solve True Crimes*. Pleasantville, N.Y.: Reader's Digest Association, 2003.

McCrary, Gregg O., with Katherine Ramsland. *The Unknown Darkness: Profiling the Predators Among Us*. New York: Harper Collins, 2003.

Morrison, Helen, and Harold Goldberg. *My Life Among the Serial Killers: Inside the Minds of the World's Most Notorious Murders*. New York: Harper Collins, 2004.

Newton, Michael. *The Encyclopedia of Serial Killers: A Study of the Chilling Criminal Phenomenon from the "Angels of Death" to the "Zodiac" Killer.* New York: Checkmark Books, 2006.

Owen, David. *Hidden Evidence: Forty True Crimes and How Forensic Science Helped Solve Them.* Buffalo, N.Y.: Firefly Books, 2009.

Phillips, Charles, and Alan Axelrod. *Cops, Crooks, and Criminologists: An International Biographical Dictionary of Law Enforcement.* New York: Checkmark Books, 2000.

Ramsland, Katherine. *The Criminal Mind: A Writer's Guide to Forensic Psychology.* Cincinnati: Writer's Digest Books, 2002.

Schechter, Harold. *The Serial Killer Files: The Who, What, Where, How, and Why of the World's Most Terrifying Murders.* New York: Random House, 2003.

Wrightsman, Lawrence S. *Forensic Psychology.* Belmont, Calif.: Wadsworth/ Thomas Learning, 2008.

For More Information

International Association of Forensic Criminologists
www.profiling.org

American Academy of Forensic Sciences
www.aafs.org

Canadian Psychological Association
www.cpa.ca

Court TV's Crime Library
www.trutv.com/library/crime/index.html

Crime and Clues: The Art and Science of Criminal Investigation
www.crimeandclues.com

FBI Academy's Behavioral Sciences Unit
www.fbi.gov/about-us/training/bsu

Federal Bureau of Investigation (FBI)
www.fbi.gov

Forensic Solutions
www.corpus-delicti.com

Institute of Behavioral Sciences
www.colorado.edu/ibs/

Society for Police and Criminal Psychology
psychweb.cisat.jmu.edu/spcp

University of Toronto's Centre for Criminology
www.criminology.utoronto.ca

U.S. Department of Justice
www.usdoj.gov

Publisher's note:
The websites listed on these pages were active at the time of publication. The publisher is not responsible for websites that have changed their addresses or discontinued operation since the date of publication. The publisher will review and update the website list upon each reprint.

Index

Picture Credits

Artville: pp. 19, 47, 58, 60, 78, 88, 101

Benjamin Stewart: p. 87

Brand-X: pp. 10, 26, 91

Corbis: pp. 37, 40

Photos.com: pp. 15, 16, 22, 29, 33, 39, 42, 51, 62, 66, 68, 72, 82, 84, 98

To the best knowledge of the publisher, all other images are in the public domain. If any image has been inadvertently uncredited, please notify Vestal Creative Services, Vestal, New York 13850, so that rectification can be made for future printings.

Biographies

AUTHOR

Joan Esherick is a full-time author, freelance writer, and professional speaker who lives outside of Philadelphia, Pennsylvania. Joan has contributed dozens of articles to national print periodicals, written spiritual and educational books, and speaks nationwide.

SERIES CONSULTANTS

Carla Miller Noziglia is Senior Forensic Advisor for the U.S. Department of Justice, International Criminal Investigative Training Assistant Program. A Fellow of the American Academy of Forensic Sciences, Ms. Noziglia served as chair of the board of Trustees of the Forensic Science Foundation. Her work has earned her many honors and commendations, including Distinguished Fellow from the American Academy of Forensic Sciences (2003) and the Paul L. Kirk Award from the American Academy of Forensic Sciences Criminalistics Section. Ms. Noziglia's publications include *The Real Crime Lab* (coeditor, 2005), *So You Want to be a Forensic Scientist* (coeditor, 2003), and contributions to *Drug Facilitated Sexual Assault* (2001), *Convicted by Juries, Exonerated by Science: Case Studies in the Use of DNA* (1996), and the *Journal of Police Science* (1989). She is on the editorial board of the *Journal for Forensic Identification*.

Jay Siegel is Director of the Forensic and Investigative Sciences Program at Indiana University-Purdue University, Indianapolis and Chair of the Department of Chemistry and Chemical Biology. He holds a Ph.D. in Analytical Chemistry from George Washington University. He worked for three years at the Virginia Bureau of Forensic Sciences, analyzing drugs, fire residues, and trace evidence. From 1980 to 2004 he was professor of forensic chemistry and director of the forensic science program at Michigan State University in the School of Criminal Justice. Dr. Siegel has testified over 200 times as an expert witness in twelve states, Federal Court and Military Court. He is editor in chief of the *Encyclopedia of Forensic Sciences*, author of *Forensic Science: A Beginner's Guide and Fundamentals of Forensic Science*, and he has more than thirty publications in forensic science journals. Dr. Siegel was awarded the 2005 Paul Kirk Award for lifetime achievement in forensic science. In February 2009, he was named Distinguished Fellow by the American Academy of Forensic Sciences.